THE ROLE OF MATRIX METALLOPROTEINASE IN HUMAN BODY PATHOLOGIES

Edited by **Francesco Travascio**

The Role of Matrix Metalloproteinase in Human Body Pathologies
http://dx.doi.org/10.5772/66560
Edited by Francesco Travascio

Contributors

Rasa Liutkeviciene, Loresa Kriauciuniene, Vykintas Liutkevicius, Agne Giedraitiene, Virginija Asmoniene, Tamara Djuric, Maja Zivkovic, Pavlína Kusnierova, Leoš Pleva, Marek Pytliak, Viliam Vanik, Peter Bojčík, Hsiao-Ming Chao, Wen-Jin Chao, Ing-Ling Chen, Xiuli Wang, Guolong Zhang, Peiru Wang, Claudia Castruita De La Rosa, Idalia Garza-Veloz, Edith Cardenas-Vargas, Rodrigo Castañeda-Miranda, Luis Octavio Solis-Sanchez, Jose Manuel Ortiz-Rodriguez, Héctor Rene Vega-Carrillo, Maria Del Rosario Martinez-Blanco, Virginia Flores-Morales, Gloria Patricia Hernandez-Delgadillo, Jose Isaias Badillo-Almaráz, Margarita L Martinez-Fierro, Sabina Zurac, Alexandra Bastian, Luciana Nichita

Published by InTech
Janeza Trdine 9, 51000 Rijeka, Croatia

Publishing Process Manager Romina Skomersic
Technical Editor SPi Global
Cover InTech Design team

First published December, 2017
Printed in Croatia
Legal deposit, Croatia: National and University Library in Zagreb

Additional hard copies can be obtained from orders@intechopen.com

The Role of Matrix Metalloproteinase in Human Body Pathologies, Edited by Francesco Travascio
p. cm.
Print ISBN 978-953-51-3717-7
Online ISBN 978-953-51-3718-4

For EU product safety concerns:
IN TECH d.o.o., Prolaz Marije Krucifikse Kozulić 3, 51000 Rijeka, Croatia,
info@intechopen.com or visit our website at intechopen.com.

Meet the editor

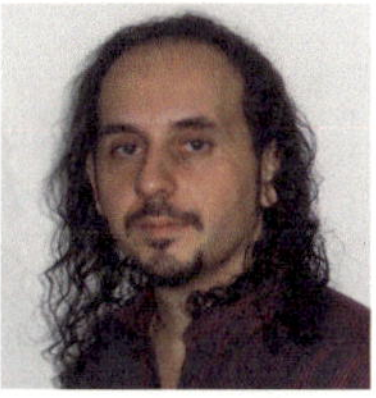

Dr. Francesco Travascio received his doctoral degree in Biomedical Engineering from the University of Miami. He is currently an assistant professor at the College of Engineering of the University of Miami, where he conducts research in the field of orthopedics at the Biomechanics Research Laboratory. In particular, Dr. Travascio investigates the mechanisms regulating the homeostasis of the extracellular matrix of cartilaginous tissues and the etiology of its degeneration with the ultimate goal of developing therapeutic approaches for tissue regeneration.

Contents

Preface

Matrix metalloproteinases (MMPs) are a family of proteolytic zinc-containing enzymes involved in physiological as well as in pathological processes in the human organism. MMPs play a key role in the remodeling of the extracellular matrix (ECM). Such a process may occur because of tissue homeostasis, morphogenesis, and tissue repair. However, remodeling could also be a part of many pathological states such as arthritis, cardiovascular diseases, neurodegenerative diseases, or impaired development in congenital anomalies. This book overviews the role of MMPs in different pathologies affecting the human body.

In particular, the role of MMPs is discussed in the context of cardiovascular diseases. MMPs play a fundamental role in remodeling cardiac ECM in both normal and pathological conditions. Changes in bioavailability of MMPs lead to pathological remodeling patterns that may eventually lead to acute and chronic heart failure, acute coronary syndromes (restenosis), atherosclerosis, and cardiomyopathies.

Also, since MMPs are capable of degrading components of the ECM responsible for remodeling during angiogenesis, abnormal levels of these enzymes have been associated with the development of pathologies such as retinal ischemia and age-related macular degeneration (AMD). It is discussed how MMPs can degrade the basilar membrane allowing capillaries to grow beneath the retina and between retinal layers. Frequent bleeding of these capillaries causes growth of fibrous tissue, retina swelling, and, consequently, impaired vision.

In the skin, MMPs play an important role in maintaining homeostasis and various pathophysiological conditions, such as skin aging and skin cancer. Reviews are presented about research progresses on MMPs in skin aging and skin cancer, including potential therapeutic approaches based on the development of MMP-specific nontoxic inhibitors.

The process of wound healing involves MMPs: during inflammation, MMPs degrade the ECM and disintegrate the capillary membrane, so that angiogenesis and cell migration take place and the damaged tissue can remodel. The imbalance in MMPs may increase the chronicity of a wound. The role of MMPs in wound healing is discussed with special emphasis on the effects of MMP unbalance in diabetic patients.

Finally, MMPs are also implicated in ECM molecule signaling and can influence proliferation, migration, differentiation, and apoptosis of cells. Their actions and activity are regulated through different mechanisms: regulation of transcription, activation of latent MMPs, and inhibition of MMP function by tissue inhibitors of metalloproteinases. About 9 of 23 human genes encoding MMPs are located on chromosome 11. A review on genetic variations in MMPs and their association with cardiovascular and neurological diseases, as well as MMP therapeutic potential through synthetic inhibitors, is reported.

Francesco Travascio, PhD
University of Miami
Coral Gables, Florida, USA

Section 1

Overview

Chapter 1

Overview of MMP Biology and Gene Associations in Human Diseases

Tamara Djuric and Maja Zivkovic

Additional information is available at the end of the chapter

http://dx.doi.org/10.5772/intechopen.70265

Abstract

Interactions of cell with the extracellular matrix (ECM) are crucial for normal development and functioning of the human organism. By regulating ECM integrity and composition matrix metalloproteinases (MMPs) play the main role in ECM molecules signaling and influence processes such as proliferation, migration, differentiation and apoptosis. ECM remodeling is a highly regulated process. When imbalanced it could contribute to pathophysiology of many diseases. The MMPs actions and activity are regulated through different mechanisms such as regulation of transcription, activation of latent MMPs, inhibition of MMP function by tissue inhibitors of metalloproteinases. MMPs are a family of calcium- and zinc-dependent endoproteinase, which share similar structural domains, but differs in substrate specificity, cell localizations and inducibility. Genetic variations in MMPs have been associated with a number of diseases, still not all findings are reproducible. Nine of 23 human genes encoding MMPs are located in a cluster on chromosome 11, which implicate their haplotype-driven effects. They could be important mediators of disease severity and could trigger acute events. In this chapter, we will review the basics of MMP biology and the most significant associations of MMPs variations with cardiovascular and neurological diseases in humans and MMPs therapeutic potential through synthetic inhibitors.

Keywords: MMP structure, MMP activation, MMP regulation, microRNA, MMP inhibitors, genetic variations, MMP haplotype

1. Introduction

Matrix metalloproteinases (MMPs) are a family of calcium (Ca^{2+})- and zinc (Zn^{2+})-dependent proteolytic enzymes involved in physiological as well as in pathological processes in the human organism. Initially they were thought to degrade only the extracellular matrix (ECM)

components, but nowadays it is well known that they have wider substrate specificity that includes non-matrix proteins of which the vast majority are bioactive molecules. Cell-cell and cell-ECM interactions are inevitable for normal development and functioning of the organism. Various proteinases are implicated in ECM remodeling, but MMPs are playing the key role. Remodeling of the tissue is crucial for physiological processes such as development, tissue homeostasis, morphogenesis and tissue repair. It could be a part of many pathological states such as arthritis, cardiovascular diseases, neurodegenerative diseases or part of the impaired development in congenital anomalies [1–4]. By regulating ECM structure and composition, MMPs are involved in growth factor availability and are playing the main role in the function of cell surface signaling systems and in that way influence proliferation, migration, differentiation and apoptosis [5]. The importance of their role in the physiological functioning of the human organism entails strict regulation of the expression and the activity of MMPs. They are regulated through different mechanisms such as regulation of transcription, activation of latent MMPs, inhibition of MMP function by tissue inhibitors of metalloproteinases (TIMPS) and so on. There is growing evidence that genetic variations in MMPs can influence gene expression or protein activity. Nine of 23 human genes encoding MMPs are located in a cluster on chromosome 11 (11q22.2–11q22.3) [6], which implicate their haplotype-driven effects. It has been shown that MMPs are important mediators of disease severity or could trigger acute events. Since they are involved in a wide spectrum of physiological and pathological processes, there is a need for determination of their precise role in different tissue and cell-specific context as well as in different stages of disease development or progression. Only then the therapeutic potential through the development of the specific inhibitors could be accurately implemented. In this chapter, we will discuss the main structural, substrate and functional properties of MMPs and give a brief review of the genetic associations with cardiovascular, neurodegenerative diseases and congenital anomalies in humans.

2. Matrix metalloproteinases

MMPs or matrixins belongs to the large family of proteinases called metzincin superfamily. Regarding its structural characteristics metzincins are subdivided into five subgroups. Other members of this superfamily are adamalysins, including a disintegrin and metalloproteinase (ADAMs) and ADAM with thrombospondin-like motif (ADAMTS), astacins, serralysins and pappalysins [7]. MMPs are expressed as zinc-dependent endopeptidases and have a wide spectrum of biological substrates that are overlapping. There are 24 genes encoding MMPs in humans, including duplicated MMP-23 gene. So, there are 23 different MMPs in humans [8]. They were named as MMP by the International Union of Biochemistry and Molecular Biology and each member of the enzyme family was assigned by a number (MMP-1, -2, -3 etc.) [9]. All MMPs contains the Zn^{2+} binding motif, HEXXHXXGXXH, in their catalytic domain and a conserved methionine forming a 'Met-turn'; are secreted in pro-pre enzyme form; need Ca^{2+} for its stability; function at neutral pH; are inhibited by TIMPs. The MMPs can be and are classified in different ways. The most common classification is based on their substrate specificity and basic domain structure. According to these criteria MMPs are subdivided into

http://dx.doi.org/10.5772/intechopen.70265

collagenases, gelatinases, stromelysins, matrilysins and membrane type-MMPs (MT-MMPs). However, there are MMPs that do not belong to any of this group specifically so they are grouped as "others" (**Figure 1**).

2.1. Structure of MMPs

MMPs domain composition and arrangements are presented in **Figure 1**. MMPs protein contains at least three homologous domains: signal peptide responsible for protein secretion, pro-peptide domain containing a consensus cysteine-switch sequence and is needed for activation of the enzyme, catalytic domain which contains a zinc-binding consensus sequence and is responsible for the proteolytic activity.

Amino-terminal signal peptide is composed of 17–29 amino acids and is responsible for targeting the enzyme to the endoplasmic reticulum and Golgi complex and for the later excretion out of the cell. The most of the MMPs are extracellular proteins except MT-MMPs that are bound to the cell surface by a transmembrane domain or glycosylphosphatidylinositol anchor.

The next, pro-peptide domain consists of 77–87 amino acids and have conserved 'cysteine switch' motif. All MMPs except MMP-23 have this motif. The thiol group from the unpaired cysteine molecule could bind to the Zn^{2+} in the catalytic domain, making the pro-MMPs inactive [10]. After the proteolytic cleavage of the bite region of the protein (serine protease, MMPs and furin) the pro-peptide domain become destabilized and the interaction between Zn^{2+} and cysteine disrupts which turns zymogens into the active MMP form. The modification of the cysteine thiol group with physiological (oxidation) or non-physiological agents (heavy metal ions) could lead to irreversible activation of the MMP by autolysis [11].

Catalytic domain contains approximately 170 amino acids and has the highest sequence homology between the metalloproteinases. It comprises Zn^{2+} binding motif HEXXHXXGXXH and a conserved methionine, forming a 'Met-turn'. This domain contains additional Zn^{2+} and Ca^{2+} ions that maintain the three-dimensional MMP structure needed for MMPs stability and enzymatic activity [12]. MMP-2 and -9 also contains three tandem fibronectin II type repeats that are responsible for elastin and gelatin binding. Typically in MMPs, carboxy-terminal end is linked to hemopexin domain with linker peptide called 'hinge region'. Hemopexin domain consists of about 200 amino acids and modulates substrate recognition. The MMP-7, -26 and -23 do not posses hinge region and hemopexin domain. MMP-23 has a unique carboxy terminal domain rich in cysteine and an immunoglobulin-like domain after the C terminus of the catalytic domain.

2.1.1. Collagenases

There are three collagenases: interstitial collagenase (MMP-1), neutrophil collagenase (MMP-8) and collagenase 3 (MMP-13). Their main characteristic is to cleave fibrillar collagens type-I, -II and -III at the specific site of the triple helices, specifically three-fourths from the N-terminus. In that way they are making characteristic ¼ and ¾ fragments. Beyond the fibrillar collagens they also degrade a number of ECM and non-ECM substrates (**Table 1**).

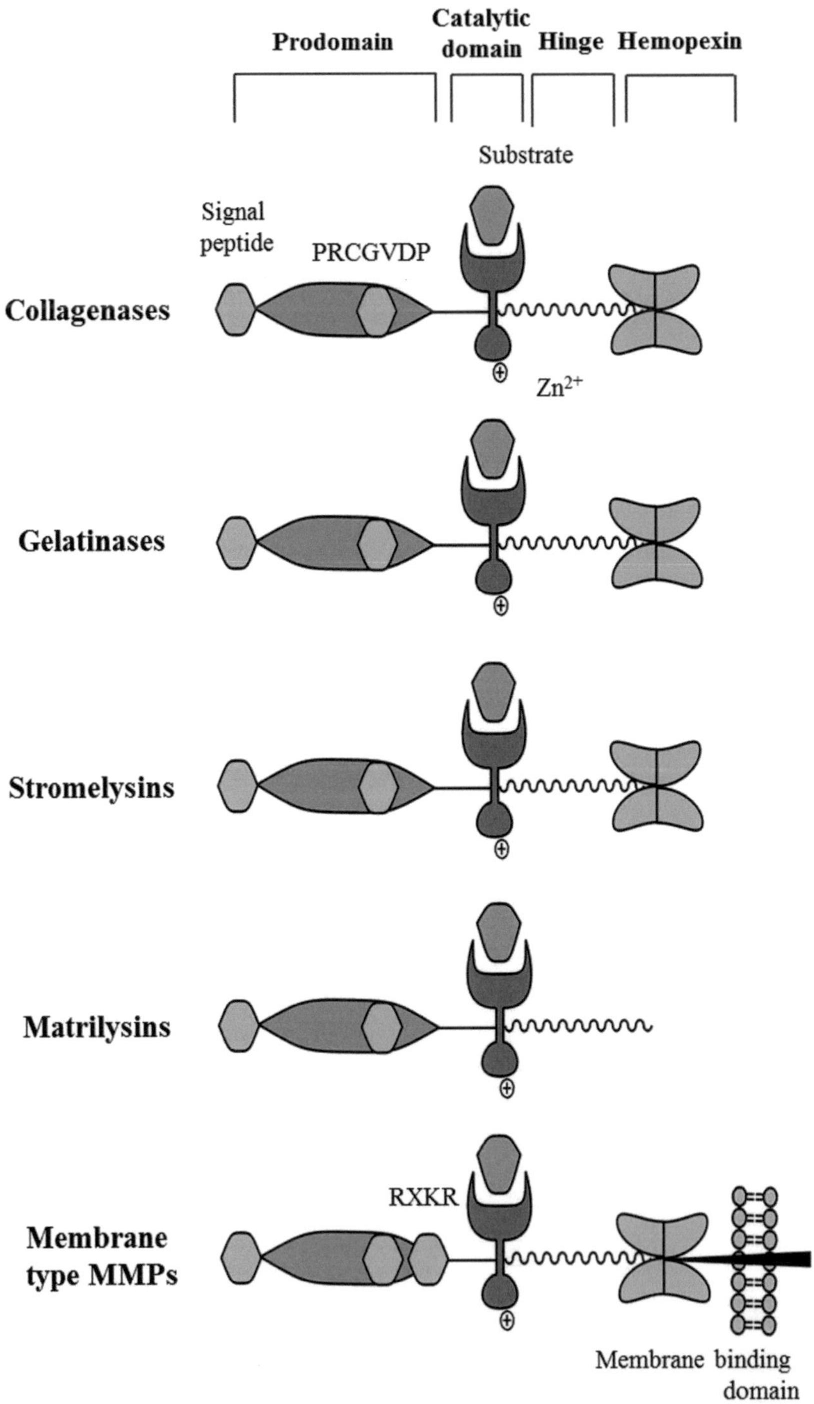

Figure 1. The domain composition and structural features of the MMPs subgroups.

MMP	Collagenous substrates	Noncollagenous ECM substrates	Non-ECM substrates
MMP-1	Collagen types I, II, III, VII, VIII, X and gelatin	Aggrecan, casein, serpins, versican, perlecan, proteoglycan link protein and tenascin-C	α1-antitrypsin/α1-antichymotrypsin, IL-1β, latent TNF-α, MCP-1,-2,-3,-4, IGFBP-2, −3, SDF-1, VEGF
MMP-2	Collagen types I, IV, V, VII, X, XI, XIV and gelatin	Aggrecan, elastin, fibronectin, laminin, perlecan, proteoglycan link protein and versican	IL-1β, Pro-IL-1β, SDF-1, MCP-3, IGFBP-3, latent TGF-β, latent TNF-α, FGFR1, pleiotrophin, CTGF
MMP-3	Collagen types II, IV, IX, X and gelatin	Aggrecan, casein, decorin, elastin, fibronectin, laminin, perlecan, proteoglycan, proteoglycan link protein and versican	α1-antitrypsin/α1-antichymotrypsin, IL-1β, Pro-IL-1β, MCP-1,-2,-3,-4, SDF-1, IGFBP-1, −3, latent TGF-β, latent TNF-α, Pro-HB-EGF, osteopontin, VEGF
MMP-7	Collagen types I, II, III, V, VI and X	Aggrecan, casein, elastin, entactin, laminin and proteoglycan link protein	α1-antitrypsin, Pro-HB-EGF, Latent TNF-α, syndecan-1, osteopontin, cellular membrane bound FasL, VEGF
MMP-8	Collagen types I, II, III, V, VII, VIII, X and gelatin	Aggrecan and laminin	α1-antitrypsin, CXCL5, IL-8
MMP-9	Collagen types V, VI, VII, X and XIV	Fibronectin, laminin, proteoglycan link protein and versican	α1-antitrypsin, IL-1β, Pro-IL-1β, CXCL5, IL-8, SDF-1, latent TGF-β, latent TNF-α, IL-2Rα, IGFBP-1, VEGF
MMP-10	Collagen types II, IV, V and gelatin	Fibronectin and laminin	
MMP-11	None known	Laminin	α1-antitrypsin, IGFBP-1
MMP-12	None known	Elastin	Latent TNF-α
MMP-13	Collagen types I, II, III, IV, V, IX, X, XI and gelatin	Aggrecan, fibronectin, laminin, perlecan and tenascin	α1-antichymotrypsin, latent TGF-β, latent TNF-α, MCP-3, SDF-1
MMP-14	Collagen types I, II, III and gelatin	Aggrecan, dermatan sulfate proteoglycan, fibrin, fibronectin, laminin, perlecan, tenascin and vitronectin	MCP-3, SDF-1
MMP-15	Collagen types I, II, III and gelatin	Aggrecan, fibronectin, laminin, perlecan, tenascin and vitronectin	
MMP-16	Collagen types I, III and gelatin	Aggrecan, casein, fibronectin, laminin, perlecan and vitronectin	VEGF
MMP-17	Gelatin	Fibrin and fibronectin	TNF-α
MMP-19	Collagen types I, IV and gelatin	Aggrecan, casein, fibronectin, laminin and tenascin	VEGF
MMP-20		Aggrecan, amelogenin and cartilage oligomeric protein	
MMP-23	Gelatin	Chondroitin sulfate, dermatan sulfate and fibronectin	

MMP	Collagenous substrates	Noncollagenous ECM substrates	Non-ECM substrates
MMP-24	Gelatin	Fibrin and fibronectin	
MMP-25	Collagen type IV and gelatin	Casein, fibrinogen and fibronectin	
MMP-26	Collagen type IV and gelatin	Casein	α1-antitrypsin
MMP-28			

MMP, matrix metalloproteinase; ECM, extracellular matrix; IL-1 interleukin 1; TNF, tumor necrosis factor; MCP, monocyte chemoattractant protein; IGFBP, Insulin-like growth factor-binding protein; SDF, stromal cell-derived factor; VEGF, vascular endothelial growth factor; TGF, tumor growth factor; FGFR, fibroblast growth factor receptor; CTGF, connective tissue growth factor; EGF, epidermal growth factor; CXCL5, C-X-C motif chemokine ligand 5; IL-8, interleukin 8; IL-2R, interleukin 2 receptor.

Table 1. MMP substrates.

2.1.2. Gelatinases

So-called gelatinase A (MMP-2) and gelatinase B (MMP-9) belongs to this group. Both of them have three repeats of a fibronectin type-II motif in the catalytic domain. They degrade denaturated collagens as well as native collagens type-IV, -V and -XI. They also denaturate gelatins, laminin and aggrecan and number of other ECM molecules. MMP-2, but not MMP-9 could cleave collagens type-I, -II and -III [13, 14]. Nevertheless, its collagenolytic activity is weaker than that of collagenases. Still, because of ability of pro-MMP-2 to recruit to the cell surface and to be activated by the MT1-MMP, it can accumulate extracellularly and have higher collagenolytic potential locally.

2.1.3. Stromelysins

Stromelysin 1 (MMP-3), stromelysin 2 (MMP-10) and stromelysin 3 (MMP-11) belongs to this group. Their name reflects the capability of degrading the wide spectrum of ECM proteins. MMP-3 and -10 degrade proteoglycans, laminin, fibronectin, vitronectin and some types of collagens but not interstitial collagens, whereas MMP-11 has a very weak affinity for ECM molecules (**Table 1**). It is located on chromosome 22, while MMP-3 and -10 are in the cluster with seven more genes on the chromosome 11 [6]. MMP-3 has the highest proteolytic efficiency in the group and is capable of activating many other pro-MMPs. It plays the main role in full activation of pro-MMP-1 [15].

2.1.4. Matrylisins

The main characteristic of matrylisins is that they lack hemopexin domain. MMP-7 and -26 belongs to this group. Both of them degrade ECM components, while MMP-7 degrade some of the cell surface molecules such as E cadherin, pro-tumor necrosis factor alpha, Fas ligand, syndecan 1 and pro-alpha defensin.

2.1.5. *Membrane-type MMPs*

There are six MT-MMPs that are divided into two groups: MMP-14, -15, -16 and -24 belongs to the type-I transmembrane proteins, while MMP-17 and MMP-25 are glycosylphosphatidylinositol-anchored proteins. All of them have a furin-like proprotein convertase recognition sequence and are activated intracellularly. All, but MT4-MMP, can activate pro-MMP2 [16]. They degrade ECM molecules, whereas MT1-MMP14 can cleave collagen type-I, -II and -III [17] and can activate proMMP-13 on the cell surface [18].

2.1.6. *Other MMPs*

Seven MMPs belong to this group. Three of them (MMP-12, -20 and -27) have a similar domain arrangement and are part of the cluster of nine genes on the chromosome 11 [6]. MMP-12 is called metalloelastase. It is mainly produced in macrophages [19] but has been found in hypertrophic chondrocytes [20] and osteoclasts [21], as well. Besides elastin it degrades other ECM proteins and is essential for macrophage migration [22]. MMP-19 is expressed in human tissues [23] and degrades basement membrane as well as other ECM molecules [24]. It is involved in tissue remodeling and migration of epithelial cells by degrading laminin 5 gamma 2 chain [25]. MMP-20, enamelysin is expressed in newly formed tooth and degrades amelogenin [26]. A mutation in this gene causes genetic disorder called amelogenin imperfecta [27]. MMP-21 is expressed in human tissues. It was found in basal and squamous cell carcinomas [28]. Annotation of its action toward ECM molecules is still not known. MMP-23 is different from other MMPs because it lacks the cysteine switch motif in the prodomain and the hemopexin domain. It posses a cysteine-rich domain which is followed by an immunoglobulin-like domain. It is mainly expressed in reproductive tissues [29]. MMP-27 is expressed in B lymphocytes [30], but the function of this enzyme in mammals is not known, yet. MMP-28, or epilysin, is expressed in many human tissues [31]. It is involved in wound repair [32] and its expression was elevated in patients with osteoarthritis [33] and rheumatoid arthritis [34]. MMP-28 overexpression up-regulated MT-MMP1 and MMP-9 in A549 lung adenocarcinoma cells [35].

2.2. Regulation of MMPs

Since they have the potential to degrade ECM and wide spectrum of non-ECM substrates and to activate other MMPs or release growth factors, matrix metalloproteinases have been stringently regulated at different levels. They are regulated at a transcriptional and translational level, by activation of the zymogen forms, by the extracellular or endogenous inhibitors, by subcellular or extracellular localization and internalization by endocytosis.

Cellular expression of MMPs is based on successive activation of multiple signaling pathways leading to synergistic effects of more transcriptional factors on the MMP promoter. Some of the most important are NF-κB, activating protein (AP)-1 and Sp-1. Recent studies have shown that endogenous miRNAs are able to recognize complementary genomic sites within human gene promoters, and in that way regulate gene transcription [36, 37]. There are multiple factors that can trigger different signaling pathways modulating MMP gene expression. They could be cytokines, chemokines or growth factors such as Interleukin-1 (IL-1), Interleukin-6 (IL-6), tumor necrosis factor alpha (TNF-α), epidermal growth factor (EGF) and platelet-derived growth factor (PDGF). The expression could also be modulated by reactive oxygen species,mechanical injury, shear or tensile stress, contact with cell bound ligands, etc. The expression of MMPs could be down-regulated by the anti inflammatory molecules such as nitric oxide (NO), transforming growth factor beta (TGF-β), Interleukin-4 (IL-4), Interleukin-10 (IL-10), interferon-γ and peroxisome proliferator-activated receptor (PPAR) (reviewed in Ref. [38]). The cell-cell and cell-matrix interactions established through adhesion molecules or integrins also have an impact on the MMPs expression [39]. Transcription could be also modified by genetic variation within the MMPs gene promoters. In the past two decades, the SNPs identified in the promoter of the MMP-1, -2, -3, -7, -9, -12, and -13 genes has been denoted as functional and associated with cardiovascular disease phenotypes (reviewed in Ref. [40]).

2.2.1. *Activation of MMPs*

Almost all MMPs are secreted as an inactive form. One of the mechanism of activation is, earlier mentioned, a 'cysteine switch' mechanism where the thiol group of the unpaired cysteine is replaced by the water. This mechanism is the first step of the stepwise activation process. It enables further pro-peptide hydroxylation of partially activated MMP or other proteases until the final step of its removal and activation [41]. Most of the MMPs are activated after the secretion, extracellularly. But the MT-MMPs and MMP-11, -23 and -28 are activated intracellularly. They have a furin recognition sequence that allows them to be activated in the Golgi apparatus by pro-protein convertase within the secretory pathway [42–45]. One of the most significant activator of MMPs in vivo is considered to be a serine protease plasmin [46]. It is shown that it activates MMP-1, -3, -7, -8, -9, -10 and -13 [46]. Other serine proteases such as mast cell proteases, chymases and tryptases also have the potential to activate pro-MMPs. Human tryptase could activate pro-MMP-3 and pro-MMP-1 but the activation of the latter is dependent on the activation of the former [47, 48].

Moreover, once activated MMPs are able to activate other pro-MMPs. For example, MMP-3 could activate pro-MMP-1, -7, -8, -9 and -13. Then, activated MMP-7 could activate zymogens pro-MMP-1, -9 and -13. Pro-MMP-2 and -3 could be activated by MMP-12 as well, while MMP-2 can activate pro-MMP-9. So, a very complex network of positive feedback loops exist and it could trigger proteolytic cleavage of the complete ECM (**Figure 2**). That is why the strict and multilevel regulation of MMPs must exist for the physiological functioning of the human organism. Inactive form of MMP-2 has somewhat specific activating mechanism which involves MT1-MMP and TIMP-2 [49]. Long story short, low or moderate levels of TIMP-2 activate pro-MMP-2 while higher levels saturate MT1-MMP and in that way inhibit activation of pro-MMP-2 [50]. Also, it was shown that other MT-MMPs (MT2-MMP, MT3-MMP, MT5-MMP and MT6-MMP) can activate pro-MMP-2 as well [51, 52]. Agents that do not have proteolytic feature, but could activate pro-MMPs, are a thiol group modifying agents oxidized glutathione and reactive oxygen species [53].

2.2.2. *microRNA and MMP*

In the last decade the novelty in the research has emphasized the role of microRNAs (miRNAs) on posttranscriptional regulation of the expression. The number of studies that have focused

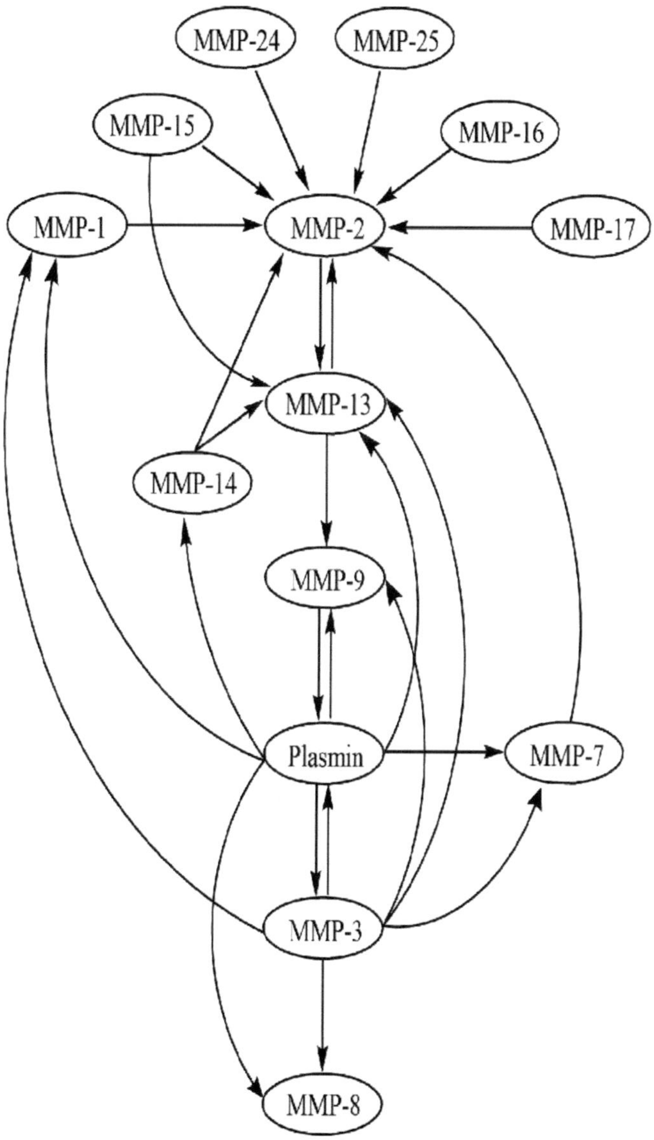

Figure 2. Mutual activation of MMPs.

on this step of MMPs regulation is growing. In this chapter, we will briefly discuss the most recent studies.

Since MMPs have an important role in the progression, metastatic potential and aggressiveness of the cancer, numerous studies have analyzed the MMP regulation by miRNAs in this disease. A recent study has investigated miRNA-489 effect on migration and invasion of hepatocellular carcinoma (HCC) cells. They have found that miRNA-489 overexpression reduced the expressions of MMP7 mRNA and protein. Additionally, miRNA-489 overexpression decreased the luciferase activity of wild type MMP7 3′-UTR but not mutated MMP7 3′-UTR in

HEK293T and HCCLM3 cells. The following rescue experiments suggest that miR-489 inhibits the migration and invasion of HCC cells, possibly by targeting MMP7 [54]. Another study has analyzed the functional background of miRNA-204-5p association with better prognosis in patients with melanoma. miRNA-204-5p is down-regulated in melanoma tissues and cells, and confers a protective effect that improves the prognosis of those patients. The binding sites of miRNA-204-5p matched the 3′-UTR of MMP-9. Up-regulation of miRNA-204-5p led to a decrease in the expression of endogenous MMP-9 and their correlation was negative. The authors have demonstrated that MMP-9 is the functional target of miRNA-204-5p in melanoma and concluded that miRNA-204-5p inhibits melanoma growth in vivo by regulating the expression of MMP-9 [55]. Using computational algorithm programs and chromatin immunoprecipitation datasets, Zheng et al. identified neighboring binding sites of myeloid zinc finger 1 (MZF1) and miRNA-337-3p within the MMP-14 promoter. They have found higher MZF1 and MMP-14 levels in gastric cancer cell lines compared to normal gastric epithelial cells. Their research results indicated that miRNA-337-3p significantly decreased the growth, invasion and angiogenesis of gastric cancer cells through repressing MZF1-facilitated MMP-14 expression in vitro, as well as in vivo on animal model [56]. Esophageal squamous cell carcinoma (ESCC) is one of the most aggressive cancers with very poor 5 year survival rate. The research has revealed that miRNA-375 is downregulated in several types of ESCC and that ectopic expression of miRNA-375 suppressed cancer cell aggressiveness in several types of cancer cells. The authors have shown significantly upregulated expression of MMP-13 in 25 ESCC specimens and ESCC cell lines compared with that in 13 normal specimens. They revealed that MMP-13 is directly regulated by antitumor miRNA-375 and acts to regulate several cell cycle promoting genes having the role in the ESCC aggressiveness [57].

With regard to the cardiovascular phenotypes a recent study has investigated miRNA-516a-5p in vascular smooth muscle cells (VSMCs) explant cultured from human abdominal aortic tissues. They have generated stable overexpression and knockdown of miRNA-516a-5p in those VSMCs. The relative MMP-2 protein expression in VSMCs with miRNA-516a-5p-overexpression was significantly higher than that in control VSMCs while the TIMP-1 levels were significantly lower. When miRNA-516a-5p was knockdowned, the opposite results were seen. Additionally, the changes in protein expression of collagen type I alpha 1 chain (COL1A1), TIMP-2 and MMP-9 have not been observed in VSMC. The authors suggested that miRNA-516a-5p may regulate MMP-2 and TIMP-1 expressions in human VSMCs, possibly promoting the proteolytic degradation of elastin for abdominal aortic aneurysm formation. [58]. Another study showed that shear-sensitive miRNA-181b binds to the TIMP-3 3′-UTR and downregulates it when overexpressed in human aortic valve endothelial cells. Additionally, it increases gelatinase/MMP activity. Through specific rescue of TIMP-3, they have clearly shown that the decreased matrix degradation results from anti-miRNA-181b treatment [59]. The miRNA-155 has been considered to be a pro-inflammatory agent, because its major target is the suppressor of cytokine signaling-1(SOCS1). It has been linked to pro-atherogenic processes in humans, as well. A recent study has shown that the SNP in the angiotensin II receptor type 1 AT1R 3′-UTR has significantly changed the miRNA-155 expression in human carotid plaques whereas rare allele homozygotes has a significantly higher expression compared to the subjects carrying wild type allele containing genotypes [60]. Also, miRNA-155 has been reported to participate in cell migration and transformation, but its function in skin wound healing was unknown. Jang et al. have been investigating the function of miRNA-155 on keratinocytes in wound healing. The results of the study showed that the protein level of MMP-2 significantly increased after miRNA-155 overexpression, while the level of TIMP-1 obviously decreased, whereas the levels of MMP-9 and TIMP-2 did not change. The authors concluded that miRNA-155 induced acceleration of keratinocyte migration is mediated at least partly through MMP-2/TIMP-1 pathway in the process of wound healing [61].

2.2.3. *Tissue inhibitors of matrix metalloproteinases (TIMPs)*

There are a lot of physiological inhibitors of MMPs in the organism. However, in tissues they are primarily regulated by TIMPs that bind MMPs in a 1:1 stoichiometry. Four mammalian TIMPs have been revealed and characterized. They are named TIMP-1, -2, -3 and -4 [62–65]. TIMP-1 and -3 are glycoproteins, while TIMP-2 and -4 do not contain carbohydrates. TIMPs inhibit all MMPs but TIMP-1 is a poor inhibitor of three membrane-type MMPs (MT1-MMP, MT3-MMP and MT5-MMP) and MMP-19 [66].

TIMPs have an N-terminal domain of approximately 125 and C-terminal domain of 65 amino acids. Both of these domains contain three conserved disulfide bonds [67, 68]. It is thought that the N-terminal domain is responsible for their binding to MMPs [67]. But there are some exceptions, C-terminal domain of TIMP-1 is shown to bind pro-MMP-9 [69]. Certain TIMPs inhibit different MMPs better than other TIMPs. Additionally, TIMPs do not inhibit only matrixins, several studies have shown that they can inhibit adamalysins as well [70, 71]. It has been shown that expression of TIMP-1 and -3 could be regulated by cytokines and growth factors such as: IL-1, fibroblast growth factor 2, platelet-derived growth factor BB, tumor growth factor-beta and tumor necrosis factor-alpha [72, 73].

TIMPs exert other functions except inhibition of MMPs. For example TIMP-1 and -2 have mitogenic activity for different type of cells [74, 75] and both have antiapoptotic activity [76, 77], while TIMP-3 has proapoptotic activity in tumor cells [78]. Solely, TIMP-2 is shown to have antiangiogenic activity [79].

Several other molecules have been reported to inhibit different MMP-s. The serpine family member, alpha2-macrogobulin, can irreversibly inhibit active MMPs in the circulation [80]. Secreted form of beta-amyloid precursor protein can inhibit MMP-2 [81]. Reversion-inducing cysteine-rich protein with Kazal motif (RECK), a GPI-anchored glycoprotein inhibits MMP-2, MMP-9 and MT1-MMP [82].

3. Synthetic MMP inhibitors

The first efforts in developing synthetic MMPs inhibitors were based on a peptide sequence recognition of the desired MMP and introduction of the group that chelated its catalytic Zn^{2+} ion. This first generation of the MMP inhibitors was called hydroxamate-based MMP inhibitors. Despite the promising results in animal models regarding their antitumor effects [83–85], following clinical studies were unsuccessful [86, 87]. The major concern was unselectivity in MMPs inhibition and serious side effects. It became clear that the knowledge of the MMPs activity in different stages of the disease and spatio-temporal expression needs to be followed in future development of the synthetic inhibitors of MMPs. Nevertheless, although hydroxamate-based MMP inhibitors have not shown the desirable effects the efforts toward their improvement had continued.

The second type of the MMP inhibitors that were developed are non-hydroxamate MMP inhibitors. The hydroxamate was replaced with other Zn^{2+} binding groups that were more metabolically stable and had higher specificity for MMPs alone. But, again the results were not satisfactory, they all had side effects in different stages of trials. From the other hand, tetracycline antibiotics have an innate ability to inhibit MMPs. The only inhibitor approved by the US Food and Drug Administration for any human disease is collagenase inhibitor doxycycline hyclate, which is a tetracycline analogue [88].

The new approach in synthetic inhibitor development has focused on targeting less conserved sites in MMPs compared to the catalytic one. This should enable more specific targeting and reduce off-target effects that the clinical trials have shown so far. As a result, inhibitors with a much stronger inhibition capacity of target MMPs have been developed [89].

The next alternative strategy has focused on the use of specific antibody fragments. Up to date, functional blocking antibodies that specifically target MT-MMPs have been developed. What is the most important, it seems that antibodies could target specific function of MMP rather than its broad proteolytic activity [90].

Part of the research has investigated the use of endogenous MMP inhibitors as potential therapeutics [91]. Nowadays, it is known that TIMPs have many of non-MMPs functions in the organism and it is very difficult to make them selective and specific to the target MMP inhibition. It could be hard to keep the balance between MMPs and TIMPs which could have serious impact on the overall MMPs activities.

So, there are few important issues to be solved before the efficacious metalloproteinase inhibitors could be made. First of all, there is a need for knowledge of precise MMP functioning and activity in cells, tissues and different stages of the disease. Also, their function in maintaining the tissue and cell homeostasis should be analyzed in details. An additional concern is their overlapping expression patterns and successive activation as well as context-dependent functioning. It seems that they could be good therapeutics for many of diseases, but the designing criteria for synthetic inhibitors are very demanding. We should combine refined and validated experimental and theoretical knowledge in order to raise the selectivity and specificity of the inhibitors toward target MMPs. Another important issue is administration of synthetic MMP inhibitors in order to avoid unnecessary toxicity of the inhibitors in the circulation. It would be of interest to determine the location (cells, tissue and organ) and temporal framework of the adverse MMP activity and develop site-specific delivery systems (detailed review in [92]).

4. MMP genes in human disease

The functions of MMPs are implicated in a variety of diseases, including those of respiratory system, central nervous system, liver, kidneys, muscles, and joints as well as the cardiovascular system [93]. Accordingly, genetic variations in genes that codes for MMPs were investigated in many of them, but only the limited number of genetic variations was thoroughly investigated. Herein, we will review mainly the findings of the genetic influence of MMPs in coronary artery disease (CAD), atherosclerosis and neurodegenerative disease.

4.1. Genetic association of variants in MMPs with vascular disease

Among all the MMPs genes only few were repeatedly investigated in a gene candidate association studies. In the year of 1996 and 1999, the two papers that investigated the functional role of promoter variants in MMP-3 [94] and MMP-9 [95] gene were published, respectively. Since then, the most investigated genetic variants in any of the MMP gene have been the MMP-3 5A/6A (rs3025058) and MMP-9-1562 C/T (rs3918242) variant, based on their role to influence gene transcription.

4.1.1. MMP-3

The common 5A/6A (rs3025058) variant in the promoter of the MMP-3 gene has been shown to affect the level of gene expression in both in vitro [94] and in vivo [96] conditions. The 5A allele was associated with higher and the 6A allele with lower transcriptional activity [94, 96]. In general, the 6A allele was mostly associated with stenosis and coronary disease progression. It was associated with greater progression of coronary artery disease (CAD) in men [97, 98] and women [99] and with the greater number of coronary arteries with significant stenosis [100, 101], but not with susceptibility to coronary heart disease [100, 102]. The 6A/6A genotype was associated with greater progression of coronary atherosclerosis [97] and the number of coronary arteries with stenosis >50% [100]. Also, it was associated with carotid stenosis >70% [103] and greater intima-media thickness (IMT) [103–105]. One or more 6A alleles had significantly higher risk for development of carotid atherosclerosis compared to 5A/5A homozygotes [106]. Besides its association with definite cardiovascular phenotypes the 5A/6A polymorphism has been linked to their risk factors such as elevated blood pressure [107], stiffer large arteries [108] and, in combination with angiotensin I-converting enzyme DD genotype, with hypertension in men [109]. On the contrary, the 5A allele as the high activity allele was predominantly associated with acute clinical events such as plaque rupture and consequently myocardial infarction (MI) [100, 110, 111]. The combination of MMP-9 and MMP-3 genotypes was found to be potentially significant for presentation of atherosclerosis. Patients with "high activity genotypes" of both SNPs had larger area of complicated atherosclerotic lesions compared to other genotypes [112]. One of the first meta-analysis that aimed to realize the effect of MMP variants on atherosclerosis found significant effect of the 5A allele on acute MI [113]. The newer meta-analysis of 15 studies (10,061 cases, 8048 controls) in coronary disease displayed no significant overall risk of coronary disease for the carriers of the 5A allele and 6A/6A genotype of rs3025058 [114]. Similarly, the haplotype-tagging approach for several SNPs (rs522616, rs650108, rs569444 and rs635746) and rs3025058 did not show significant difference in genotype distribution in MI patients compared to controls [114]. The meta-analysis of 8 SNPs selected from the studies in which 58 SNPs within MMPs and TIMPs were investigated in abdominal aortic aneurism (AAA) pinpoint the significant association of only MMP-3 rs3025058 with AAA presence [115]. Another one, published the same year, which was investigated several genes in AAA presented the similar results for MMP-3 rs3025058 [116].

4.1.2. MMP-9

The first main role of MMP-9, which gave the rationale for the investigation in aterogenesis is the degradation of basement membrane, which surrounds each VSMC and is primarily composed of type-IV collagen, laminin and fibronectin [117]. The MMP-9 gene possesses several single nucleotide polymorphisms, the most widely studied of which is the −1562 C/T gene polymorphism (rs3918242) in the promoter of the MMP-9 gene [118]. It was suggested that this polymorphism has a functional capacity to regulate MMP-9 expression, since luciferase reporter assays showed higher promoter activity of the T allele in vitro [95]. Although in this study authors have not found the significant effect of the rare allele on the susceptibility to MI they suggested its role in coronary artery severity [95]. Recently, another study challenged the functional role of this SNP [119]. In cells with different −1562C/T genotypes there was neither difference in MMP-9 expression level nor in MMP-9 promoter activity [119]. Nevertheless, this variant was extensively and repeatedly studied in CAD. Both positive [120, 121] and negative [122, 123] association of −1562T allele with the disease were presented. The meta-analysis of previous studies showed no association of MMP-9-1562 C/T polymorphism with coronary heart disease [113]. The other one, which included 11 polymorphisms from MMPs showed that Glu45Lys in MMP3 gene and −1562C/T in MMP9 gene had an overall significant association with CAD [124]. In one of the biggest gene association studies of MMP genes in MI and CAD the composite genotypes of MMP-9 variations CT/RQ had greater risk for MI after full adjustment for covariates [125].

Arterial stiffness and MMP-9 levels were explored in healthy subjects in association with common risk factors and MMP-9 variations. Mean aortic pulse wave velocity (PWV) values were significantly higher in the carriers of the 1562 T and 279 Q alleles compared with common homozygotes, as well as serum MMP-9 levels [126]. The rs3918242 and exon 6 R279Q A/G (rs17576) polymorphisms were not associated with the presence of CAD or MI, but R279Q was associated with hypertension [127]. Among several MMP-2, MMP-7 and MMP-9 variations the MMP-9 R668Q genetic variant was associated with left ventricular dysfunction [128].

In order to overcome a simplistic mechanistic interpretation of the −1562T allele roles in regulation of MMP-9 gene expression, the five promoter and nine exon SNPs, which change amino acid in the encoded protein, were analyzed. The functional consequences of these SNPs were investigated [129]. Three exon SNPs altered the specific enzymatic activity while altered promoter activity was shown for four promoter SNPs among which was the −1562C/T [129]. Still, for promoter SNPs the explanation of how they exert their effect is not known, yet.

Recently, several variants in the 3′ UTR of the MMP-9 gene were analyzed in association with atherosclerotic cerebral infarction (ACI) in Chinese population. They found a significant association of the rare C allele and CC genotype of rs1056628 with ACI. Also the haplotype rs20544C-rs1056628C-rs9509T showed significantly increased risk for ACI. Further findings indicated that miR-491 directly targets MMP-9 and that the A–C transition in rs1056628, which is located in the miR-491 seed sequence, could influence the miR-491 binding. Moreover, the miR-491 decreased MMP-9 protein expression in cotransfected HUVEC, but did not show the influence on the mRNA expression [130].

4.1.3. MMP-2

The other gelatinase, MMP-2, contrary to MMP-9 is constitutively expressed in many of the connective tissue cells that have a role in the vascular system. It is also functionally implicated in the processes of cell invasion, migration of smooth muscle cells (SMC) and destabilization of atherosclerotic plaque. The 15 novel sequence variants in the MMP-2 gene were firstly described in the year of 2001 [131] among which six were in the promoter of the gene and six in the coding region. Among three promoter variants that map onto cis-acting elements the one that disrupts SP-1 type of promoter site (−1306 C/T, rs243865) showed the lower promoter activity in rare allele [131]. The −790 T allele was associated with triple vessel disease [132].

4.1.4. MMP-1

Similarly to other MMP genes the study of MMP-1 genetic variants started with a definition of potentially functional SNPs. First, the 2G-allele of −1607 1G/2G variation in the MMP-1 promoter has been noted to increase transcriptional activity by creating an E26 transcription factor binding site [133]. Next, in vitro analysis in human macrophages showed that the A–519-C–340 and G–519-T–340 haplotypes compared with the A–519-T–340 haplotype, had lower promoter activity, whereas the G–519-C–340 haplotype had greater promoter strength [134]. At the same time that study was one of the first which investigated the genetic variations in MMP-1, solely and in haplotype, in association with cardiovascular disease. It revealed both, risk (G–519-C–340) and protective (A–519-C–340 and G–519-T–340) MMP-1 haplotypes in MI [134]. Recently, the −340 T/C, −519 A/G and −1607 1G/2G variations, separately and in haplotype were associated with the occurrence of carotid plaques (CP). Compared to the referent haplotype 2G–1607-T–340-A–519, the haplotypes 1G–1607-T–34-A–519, 1G–1607-T–340-G–519 and 2G–1607-C–340-A–519 had statistically significant protective effect on CP presence. The MMP-1–1607 2G allele had significantly increased allele dose-dependent risk for CP presence [2]. Previously, the 2G allele also appeared to favor carotid artery stenosis [103].

SNPs in genes encoding MMP-1, -2, -3 and -9 and TIMP-1, -2 and -3 were associated with MI and CAD and combinations of MMP-1 1G/2G and MMP-3 5A/6A genotypes were significantly associated with CAD, but not MI [125]. Recently, the MMP-1/MMP-3 less active haplotype 1G–1607-6A was described as a significant risk factor for obstructive uropathy, which is characterized by collagen accumulation [4]. Others did not find the association of the selected SNPs in MMP1, MMP2, MMP3, MMP9 or MMP10 with either acute MI compared with angina, or with coronary disease compared with controls [135]. Recently, the genome-wide association analysis was performed using 500 K SNPs to identify genes influencing variation in serum levels of MMP-1 [136]. The cluster of 179 SNPs in the cluster on chromosome 11 were associated with MMP-1 serum levels, with the peak of association on rs495366, which is located between the MMP-1 and MMP-3 genes [136].

4.1.5. MMP-8

The investigation of the genetic variations in MMP-8 started with the identification of several polymorphisms in the MMP8 gene, at −799 C/T (rs11225395), −381 A/G (rs1320632) and +17 C/G. Their functional capacity was suggested after the study showed significantly higher promoter activity of the construct that contained the minor alleles compared to the construct with major alleles [137]. Many of the forthcoming studies investigated the role of MMP-8 in atherosclerosis. After analysis of selected 16 SNPs in the MMP-8 gene the rs1940475, in the coding region of the MMP-8 gene, was associated with the extent of coronary atherosclerosis [138]. Also, the minor T allele of rs1940475 was associated with a protective effect against carotid atherosclerosis progression in a 10-year follow-up [138]. In another study the significantly higher frequency of the −381 G allele was found in female patients with carotid atherosclerosis compared to controls [139]. The significantly higher expression of MMP-8 mRNA was found in carotid plaques of the G−381 T−799 haplotype compared to the reference A−381C−799 haplotype [139].

One of the not so commonly investigated MMP gene, the MMP 14, was significantly associated with ultrasonographically defined plaque phenotype suggesting protective effect of rs2236307 major T allele for vulnerable plaque, in Chinese Han population [140].

It seems that a precise definition of particular phenotypes of interest is necessary to get the reproducible findings about genetic influence of a variant in complex disease. The CAD endpoints, the study design as well as a selection of the controls in association studies might influence the findings. The good example of previous is the particular meta-analysis performed for MMP family gene variants [124].

4.1.6. Serum levels of MMPs in atherosclerosis

Over the past 15 years the protein, plasma and serum levels of MMPs were investigated in association with cardiovascular and atherosclerotic plaque phenotypes (mainly MMP-1, MMP-2, MMP-9, MMP-13 and recently MMP-8). MMP-1 but not MMP-9 serum levels were associated with the total plaque burden [141]. Both, MMP-9 and MMP-8 serum and plasma levels were associated with cardiovascular outcomes in CAD patients [142–144]. Although MMP-8 cleaves collagen type-I three times more potently than two other interstitial collagenases, MMP-1 and MMP-13 [145], its role in CAD was lesser investigated in comparison to other MMPs, until recently. MMP-8 plasma levels were associated with unstable angina [146] and with the occurrence of carotid plaque [147]. Among the serum levels of MMP-1, -2, -3, -8, -9, -13, and TIMP-1, -2, -3, -4 analyzed prospectively after the MI only the baseline levels of MMP-8 were significantly associated with changes in left ventricular end-diastolic volume after the adjustment for covariates [148].

4.2. Genetics of MMPs in brain disease

In the central nervous system, MMPs have an important role and may influence proteolysis of basement membranes, extracellular matrix molecules, precursors of the cytokines, cell surface molecules and myelin components. In healthy central nervous system (CNS), they also have a role in synaptic plasticity, learning and memory. It is known that MMPs play a significant role in Alzheimer's disease (AD), Parkinson's disease (PD) and multiple sclerosis (MS). Their role in neuroinflammation and neurodegeneration was reviewed in detail in Brkic et al. [149]. Thus, as reasonable candidate genes the variations in MMPs were investigated in several neurological diseases.

The results in this field were also partly inconsistent. While one of the first studies that investigated MMP-9 polymorphism in multiple sclerosis had not found that it is a susceptibility marker for MS [150] two other studies showed the significant decrease in the MMP-9 rs3918242 rare T allele carrier ship in female patients with MS [3, 151]. The same allele was found to be more often in patients with PD and amyotrophic lateral sclerosis [152]. The haplotype formed by the −1562 T allele and the L allele ((CA)(<or = 20)) of −90 (CA)n repeat polymorphism in MMP-9 was over-represented in patients with MS in comparison to controls [153]. Others suggested that haplotypes of these two polymorphisms might modulate disease severity, expressed through expanded disability status scale (EDSS) [154]. The MMP-3 6A/6A genotype was also associated with disease severity, showing significantly higher mean multiple sclerosis severity score (MSSS) values in comparison to other genotypes [155]. In another study, the MMP-2 −1575 G/A variation was shown to influence the age of disease onset in MS patients with optic neuritis as a first symptom [156]. The four polymorphism haplotypes in the gene encoding MMP-3 was associated with changes in amyloid beta levels in non-demented subjects [157] but no evidence was found that the MMP-3gene is causally involved in dementia or AD [158].

4.3. Genetic epilogue

In the last few years the explosion of the data regarding the genetic variations and their association with disease happened as a consequence of the use of high throughput technologies, genome wide association studies, bioinformatical databases, etc. Thus, the results of the candidate gene association studies should be combined with the findings of the different genetic analysis approaches. Some of the genetic variations mentioned above cannot even be found on the arrays, as they are the insertion/deletion variation type, for example, MMP-3 5A/6A or MMP-1 1G/2G. The majority of studies that consider the role of MMPs in different pathologies did not include the genetic component, thus a lot is to be done yet in specifying the genetic architecture of MMPs in health and disease.

Author details

Tamara Djuric* and Maja Zivkovic

*Address all correspondence to: tamariska@vin.bg.ac.rs

VINCA Institute of Nuclear Sciences, Laboratory for Radiobiology and Molecular Genetics, University of Belgrade, Belgrade, Serbia

References

[1] Scherer S, de Souza TB, de Paoli J, Brenol CV, Xavier RM, Brenol JC, Chies JA, Simon D. Matrix metalloproteinase gene polymorphisms in patients with rheumatoid arthritis. Rheumatology International. 2010;**30**:369-373. DOI: 10.1007/s00296-009-0974-8

[2] Djurić T, Stojković L, Zivković M, Končar I, Stanković A, Djordjević A, Alavantić D. Matrix metalloproteinase-1 promoter genotypes and haplotypes are associated with carotid plaque presence. Clinical Biochemistry. 2012;**45**:1353-1356. DOI: 10.1016/j.clinbiochem.2012.05.032

[3] Zivković M, Djurić T, Dincić E, Raicević R, Alavantić D, Stanković A. Matrix metalloproteinase-9 −1562 C/T gene polymorphism in Serbian patients with multiple sclerosis. Journal of Neuroimmunology. 2007;**189**:147-150. DOI: 10.1016/j.jneuroim.2007.06.022

[4] Djuric T, Zivkovic M, Milosevic B, Andjelevski M, Cvetkovic M, Kostic M, Stankovic A. MMP-1 and -3 haplotype is associated with congenital anomalies of the kidney and urinary tract. Pediatric Nephrology. 2014;**29**:879-884. DOI: 10.1007/s00467-013-2699-x

[5] Egeblad M, Werb Z. New functions for the matrix metalloproteinases in cancer progression. Nature Reviews. Cancer. 2002;**2**:161-174. DOI: 10.1038/nrc745

[6] Pendas AM, Santamaria I, Alvarez MV, Pritchard M, Lopez-Otin C. Fine physical mapping of the human matrix metalloproteinase genes clustered on chromosome 11q22.3. Genomics. 1996;**37**:266-268. DOI: 10.1006/geno.1996.0557

[7] Sterchi EE. Special issue: metzincin metalloproteinases. Molecular Aspects of Medicine. 2008;**29**:255-257. DOI: 10.1016/j.mam.2008.08.007

[8] Murphy G, Nagase H. Progress in matrix metalloproteinase research. Molecular Aspects of Medicine. 2008;**29**:290-308. DOI: 10.1016/j.mam.2008.05.002

[9] Iyer RP, Patterson NL, Fields GB, Lindsey ML. The history of matrix metalloproteinases: Milestones, myths, and misperceptions. American Journal of Physiology. Heart and Circulatory Physiology. 2012;**303**:H919-H930. DOI: 10.1152/ajpheart.00577.2012

[10] Van Wart HE, Birkedal-Hansen H. The cysteine switch: A principle of regulation of metalloproteinase activity with potential applicability to the entire matrix metalloproteinase gene family. Proceedings of the National Academy of Sciences of the United States of America. 1990;**87**:5578-5582

[11] Ra HJ, Parks WC. Control of matrix metalloproteinase catalytic activity. Matrix Biology. 2007;**26**:587-596. DOI: 10.1016/j.matbio.2007.07.001

[12] Bode W, Gomis-Rüth FX, Stöckler W. Astacins, serralysins, snake venom and matrix metalloproteinases exhibit identical zinc-binding environments (HEXXHXXGXXH and met-turn) and topologies and should be grouped into a common family, the 'metzincins'. FEBS Letters. 1993;**331**:134-140. DOI: 10.1016/0014-5793(93)80312-I

[13] Aimes RT, Quigley JP. Matrix metalloproteinase-2 is an interstitial collagenase. Inhibitor-free enzyme catalyzes the cleavage of collagen fibrils and soluble native type I collagen generating the specific 3/4- and 1/4-length fragments. The Journal of Biological Chemistry. 1995;**270**:5872-5876. DOI: 10.1074/jbc.270.11.5872

[14] Patterson ML, Atkinson SJ, Knäuper V, Murphy G. Specific collagenolysis by gelatinase a, MMP-2, is determined by the hemopexin domain and not the fibronectin-like domain. FEBS Letters. 2001;**503**:158-162. DOI: 10.1016/S0014-5793(01)02723-5

[15] Suzuki K, Enghild JJ, Morodomi T, Salvesen G, Nagase H. Mechanisms of activation of tissue procollagenase by matrix metalloproteinase 3 (stromelysin). Biochemistry. 1990;**29**: 10261-10270

[16] English WR, Holtz B, Vogt G, Knäuper V, Murphy G. Characterization of the role of the "MT-loop": An eight-amino acid insertion specific to progelatinase A (MMP2) activating membrane-type matrix metalloproteinases. The Journal of Biological Chemistry. 2001;**276**:42018-42026. DOI: 10.1074/jbc.M107783200

[17] Ohuchi E, Imai K, Fujii Y, Sato H, Seiki M, Okada Y. Membrane type1 matrix metalloproteinase digests interstitial collagens and other extracellular matrix macromolecules. The Journal of Biological Chemistry. 1997;**272**:2446-2451. DOI: 10.1074/jbc.272.4.2446

[18] Knäuper V, Will H, López-Otin C, Smith B, Atkinson SJ, Stanton H, Hembry RM, Murphy G. Cellular mechanisms for human procollagenase-3 (MMP-13) activation. Evidence that MT1-MMP (MMP-14) and gelatinase a (MMP-2) are able to generate active enzyme. The Journal of Biological Chemistry. 1996;**271**:17124-17131. DOI: 10.1074/jbc.271.29.17124

[19] Shapiro SD, Kobayashi DK, Ley TJ. Cloning and characterization of a unique elastolytic metalloproteinase produced by human alveolar macrophages. The Journal of Biological Chemistry. 1993;**268**:23824-23829

[20] Kerkelä E, Bohling T, Herva R, Uria JA, Saarialho-Kere U. Human macrophage metalloelastase (MMP-12) expression is induced in chondrocytes during fetal development and malignant transformation. Bone. 2001;**29**:487-493

[21] Hou P, Troen T, Ovejero MC, Kirkegaard T, Andersen TL, Byrjalsen I, Ferreras M, Sato T, Shapiro SD, Foged NT, Delaisse JM. Matrix metalloproteinase-12 (MMP-12) in osteoclasts: New lesson on the involvement of MMPs in bone resorption. Bone. 2004; **34**:37-47

[22] Shipley JM, Wesselschmidt RL, Kobayashi DK, Ley TJ, Shapiro SD. Metalloelastase is required for macrophage-mediated proteolysis and matrix invasion in mice. Proceedings of the National Academy of Sciences of the United States of America. 1996;**93**: 3942-3946

[23] Pendas AM, Knäuper V, Puente XS, Llano E, Mattei MG, Apte S, Murphy G, López-Otín C. Identification and characterization of a novel human matrix metalloproteinase with unique structural characteristics, chromosomal location, and tissue distribution. The Journal of Biological Chemistry. 1997;**272**:4281-4286. DOI: 10.1074/jbc.272.7.4281

[24] Stracke JO, Hutton M, Stewart M, Pendas AM, Smith B, Lopez-Otin C, Murphy G, Knauper V. Biochemical characterization of the catalytic domain of human matrix metalloproteinase 19—Evidence for a role as a potent basement membrane degrading enzyme. The Journal of Biological Chemistry. 2000;**275**:14809-14816

[25] Sadowski T, Dietrich S, Koschinsky F, Ludwig A, Proksch E, Titz B, Sedlacek R. Matrix metalloproteinase 19 processes the laminin 5 gamma 2 chain and induces epithelial cell migration. Cellular and Molecular Life Sciences. 2005;**62**:870-880. DOI: 10.1007/s00018-005-4478-8

[26] Ryu OH, Fincham AG, Hu CC, Zhang C, Qian Q, Bartlett JD, Simmer JP. Characterization of recombinant pig enamelysin activity and cleavage of recombinant pig and mouse amelogenins. Journal of Dental Research. 1999;**78**:743-750

[27] Li W, Gibson CW, Abrams WR, Andrews DW, DenBesten PK. Reduced hydrolysis of amelogenin may result in X-linked amelogenesis imperfecta. Matrix Biology. 2001;**19**:755-760. DOI: 10.1016/S0945-053X(00)00121-9

[28] Ahokas K, Lohi J, Illman SA, Llano E, Elomaa O, Impola U, Karjalainen-Lindsberg ML, Saarialho-Kere U. Matrix metalloproteinase-21 is expressed epithelially during development and in cancer and is up-regulated by transforming growth factor-beta1 in keratinocytes. Laboratory Investigation. 2003;**83**:1887-1899. DOI: 10.1097/01.LAB.0000106721.86126.39

[29] Velasco G, Pendás AM, Fueyo A, Knäuper V, Murphy G, López-Otín C. Cloning and characterization of human MMP-23, a new matrix metalloproteinase predominantly expressed in reproductive tissues and lacking conserved domains in other family members. The Journal of Biological Chemistry. 1999;**274**:4570-4576. DOI: 10.1074/jbc.274.8.4570

[30] Bar-Or A, Nuttall RK, Duddy M, Alter A, Kim HJ, Ifergan I, Pennington CJ, Bourgoin P, Edwards DR, Yong VW. Analyses of all matrix metalloproteinase members in leukocytes emphasize monocytes as major inflammatory mediators in multiple sclerosis. Brain. 2003;**126**:2738-2749. DOI: 10.1093/brain/awg285

[31] Lohi J, Wilson CL, Roby JD, Parks WC. Epilysin, a novel human matrix metalloproteinase (MMP-28) expressed in testis and keratinocytes and in response to injury. The Journal of Biological Chemistry. 2001;**276**:10134-10144. DOI: 10.1074/jbc.M001599200

[32] Saarialho-Kere U, Kerkelä E, Jahkola T, Suomela S, Keski-Oja J, Lohi J. Epilysin (MMP-28) expression is associated with cell proliferation during epithelial repair. The Journal of Investigative Dermatology. 2002;**119**:14-21. DOI: 10.1046/j.1523-1747.2002.01790.x

[33] Kevorkian L, Young DA, Darrah C, Donell ST, Shepstone L, Porter S, Brockbank SM, Edwards DR, Parker AE, Clark IM. Expression profiling of metalloproteinases and their inhibitors in cartilage. Arthritis and Rheumatism. 2004;**50**:131-141. DOI: 10.1002/art.11433

[34] Momohara S, Okamoto H, Komiya K, Ikari K, Takeuchi M, Tomatsu T, Kamatani N. Matrix metalloproteinase 28/epilysin expression in cartilage from patients with rheumatoid arthritis and osteoarthritis: Comment on the article by Kevorkian et al. Arthritis and Rheumatism. 2004;**50**:4074-4075; author reply 4075. DOI: 10.1002/art.20799

[35] Illman SA, Lehti K, Keski-Oja J, Lohi J. Epilysin (MMP-28) induces TGF-beta mediated epithelial to mesenchymal transition in lung carcinoma cells. Journal of Cell Science. 2006;**119**:3856-3865. DOI: 10.1242/jcs.03157

[36] Kim DH, Sætrom P, Snøve O, Rossi JJ. MicroRNA-directed transcriptional gene silencing in mammalian cells. Proceedings of the National Academy of Sciences of the United States of America. 2008;**105**:16230-16235. DOI: 10.1073/pnas.0808830105

[37] Younger ST, Corey DR. Transcriptional gene silencing in mammalian cells by miRNA mimics that target gene promoters. Nucleic Acids Research. 2011;**39**:5682-5691. DOI: 10.1093/nar/gkr155

[38] Johnson JL. Matrix metalloproteinases: Influence on smooth muscle cells and atherosclerotic plaque stability. Expert Review of Cardiovascular Therapy. 2007;**5**:265-282. DOI: 10.1586/14779072.5.2.265

[39] Nagase H, Woessner JF Jr. Matrix metalloproteinases. The Journal of Biological Chemistry. 1999;**274**:21491-21494. DOI: 10.1074/jbc.274.31.21491

[40] Ye S. Influence of matrix metalloproteinase genotype on cardiovascular disease susceptibility and outcome. Cardiovascular Research. 2006;**69**:636-645. DOI: 10.1016/j.cardiores.2005.07.015

[41] Nagase H. Activation mechanisms of matrix metalloproteinases. Biological Chemistry. 1997;**378**:151-160

[42] Sato H, Kinoshita T, Takino T, Nakayama K, Seiki M. Activation of a recombinant membrane type 1-matrix metalloproteinase (MT1-MMP) by furin and its interaction with tissue inhibitor of metalloproteinases (TIMP)-2. FEBS Letters. 1996;**393**:101-104. DOI: 10.1016/0014-5793(96)00861-7

[43] Wang X, Pei D. Shedding of membrane type matrix metalloproteinase 5 by a furin-type convertase: A potential mechanism for down-regulation. The Journal of Biological Chemistry. 2001;**276**:35953-35960. DOI: 10.1074/jbc.M103680200

[44] Kang T, Nagase H, Pei D. Activation of membrane-type matrix metalloproteinase 3 zymogen by the proprotein convertase furin in the trans-Golgi network. Cancer Research. 2002;**62**:675-681

[45] Pei D, Weiss SJ. Furin-dependent intracellular activation of the human stromelysin-3 zymogen. Nature. 1995;**375**:244-247. DOI: 10.1038/375244a0

[46] Lijnen HR. Plasmin and matrix metalloproteinases in vascular remodeling. Thrombosis and Haemostasis. 2001;**86**:324-333

[47] Gruber BL, Marchese MJ, Suzuki K, Schwartz LB, Okada Y, Nagase H, Ramamurthy NS. Synovial procollagenase activation by human mast cell tryptase dependence upon matrix metalloproteinase 3 activation. The Journal of Clinical Investigation. 1989;**84**:1657-1662. DOI: 10.1172/JCI114344

[48] Johnson JL, Jackson CL, Angelini GD, George SJ. Activation of matrix-degrading metalloproteinases by mast cell proteases in atherosclerotic plaques. Arteriosclerosis, Thrombosis, and Vascular Biology. 1998;**18**:1707-1715. DOI: 10.1161/01.ATV.18.11.1707

[49] Sato H, Takino T, Okada Y, Cao J, Shinagawa A, Yamamoto E, Seiki M. A matrix metalloproteinase expressed on the surface of invasive tumor cells. Nature. 1994;**370**:61-65

[50] Strongin AY, Collier I, Bannikov G, Marmer BL, Grant GA, Goldberg GI. Mechanism of cell surface activation of 72-kDa type IV collagenase. Isolation of the activated form of the membrane metalloprotease. The Journal of Biological Chemistry. 1995;**270**:5331-5338. DOI: 10.1074/jbc.270.10.5331

[51] Visse R, Nagase H. Matrix metalloproteinases and tissue inhibitors of metalloproteinases: Structure, function, and biochemistry. Circulation Research. 2003;**92**:827-839. DOI: 10.1161/01.RES.0000070112.80711.3D

[52] Nie J, Pei D. Direct activation of pro-matrix metalloproteinase-2 by leukolysin/membrane-type 6 matrix metalloproteinase/matrix metalloproteinase 25 at the asn(109)-Tyr bond. Cancer Research. 2003;**63**:6758-6762

[53] Nelson KK, Melendez JA. Mitochondrial redox control of matrix metalloproteinases. Free Radical Biology & Medicine. 2004;**37**:768-784. DOI: 10.1016/j.freeradbiomed.2004.06.008

[54] Lin Y, Liu J, Huang Y, Liu D, Zhang G, Kan H. microRNA-489 plays an anti-metastatic role in human hepatocellular carcinoma by targeting matrix metalloproteinase-7. Translational Oncology. 2017;**10**:211-220. DOI: 10.1016/j.tranon.2017.01.010

[55] Luan W, Qian Y, Ni X, Bu X, Xia Y, Wang J, Ruan H, Ma S, Xu B. miR-204-5p acts as a tumor suppressor by targeting matrix metalloproteinases-9 and B-cell lymphoma-2 in malignant melanoma. OncoTargets and Therapy. 2017;**10**:1237-1246. DOI: 10.2147/OTT.S128819

[56] Zheng L, Jiao W, Mei H, Song H, Li D, Xiang X, Chen Y, Yang F, Li H, Huang K, Tong Q. miRNA-337-3p inhibits gastric cancer progression through repressing myeloid zinc finger 1-facilitated expression of matrix metalloproteinase 14. Oncotarget. 2016;**7**:40314-40328. DOI: 10.18632/oncotarget.9739

[57] Osako Y, Seki N, Kita Y, Yonemori K, Koshizuka K, Kurozumi A, Omoto I, Sasaki K, Uchikado Y, Kurahara H, Maemura K, Natsugoe S. Regulation of MMP13 by antitumor microRNA-375 markedly inhibits cancer cell migration and invasion in esophageal squamous cell carcinoma. International Journal of Oncology. 2016;**49**:2255-2264. DOI: 10.3892/ijo.2016.3745

[58] Chan CY, Cheuk BL, Cheng SW. Abdominal aortic aneurysm-associated microRNA-516a-5p regulates expressions of methylenetetrahydrofolate reductase, matrix metalloproteinase-2, and tissue inhibitor of matrix metalloproteinase-1 in human abdominal aortic vascular smooth muscle cells. Annals of Vascular Surgery. 2017;**42**:263-273.DOI: 10.1016/j.avsg.2016.10.062

[59] Heath JM, Fernandez Esmerats J, Khambouneheuang L, Kumar S, Simmons R, Jo H. Mechanosensitive microRNA-181b regulates aortic valve endothelial matrix degradation by targeting TIMP3. Cardiovascular Engineering and Technology. 2017. DOI: 10.1007/s13239-017-0296-z

[60] Stanković A, Kolaković A, Živković M, Djurić T, Bundalo M, Končar I, Davidović L, Alavantić D. Angiotensin receptor type 1 polymorphism A1166C is associated with altered

AT1R and miR-155 expression in carotid plaque tissue and development of hypoechoic carotid plaques. Atherosclerosis. 2016;**248**:132-9. DOI: 10.1016/j.atherosclerosis.2016.02.032

[61] Yang L, Zheng Z, Zhou Q, Bai X, Fan L, Yang C, Su L, Hu D. miR-155 promotes cutaneous wound healing through enhanced keratinocytes migration by MMP-2. Journal of Molecular Histology. 2017;**48**:147-155. DOI: 10.1007/s10735-017-9713-8

[62] Carmichael DF, Sommer A, Thompson RC, Anderson DC, Smith CG, Welgus HG, Stricklin GP. Primary structure and cDNA cloning of human fibroblast collagenase inhibitor. Proceedings of the National Academy of Sciences of the United States of America. 1986;**83**:2407-2411

[63] Stetler-Stevenson WG, Krutzsch HC, Liotta LA. Tissue inhibitor of metalloproteinase (TIMP-2). A new member of the metalloproteinase inhibitor family. The Journal of Biological Chemistry. 1989;**264**:17374-17378

[64] Wick M, Bürger C, Brüsselbach S, Lucibello FC, Müller R. A novel member of human tissue inhibitor of metalloproteinases (TIMP) gene family is regulated during G1 progression, mitogenic stimulation, differentiation, and senescence. The Journal of Biological Chemistry. 1994;**269**:18953-18960

[65] Greene J, Wang M, Liu YE, Raymond LA, Rosen C, Shi YE. Molecular cloning and characterization of human tissue inhibitor of metalloproteinase 4. The Journal of Biological Chemistry. 1996;**271**:30375-30380. DOI: 10.1074/jbc.271.48.30375

[66] Baker AH, Edwards DR, Murphy G. Metalloproteinase inhibitors: Biological actions and therapeutic opportunities. Journal of Cell Science. 2002;**115**:3719-3727. DOI: 10.1242/jcs.00063

[67] Murphy G, Houbrechts A, Cockett MI, Williamson RA, O'Shea M, Docherty AJ. The N-terminal domain of tissue inhibitor of metalloproteinases retains metalloproteinase inhibitory activity. Biochemistry. 1991;**30**:8097-8102

[68] Williamson RA, Marston FA, Angal S, Koklitis P, Panico M, Morris HR, Carne AF, Smith BJ, Harris TJ, Freedman RB. Disulfide bondassignment in human tissue inhibitor of metalloproteinases (TIMP). The Biochemical Journal. 1990;**268**:267-274

[69] Fassina G, Ferrari N, Brigati C, Benelli R, Santi L, Noonan DM, Albini A. Tissue inhibitors of metalloproteases: Regulation and biological activities. Clinical & Experimental Metastasis. 2000;**18**:111-120

[70] Wang WM, Ge G, Lim NH, Nagase H, Greenspan DS. TIMP-3 inhibits the procollagen N-proteinase ADAMTS-2. The Biochemical Journal. 2006;**398**:515-519. DOI: 10.1042/BJ20060630

[71] Jacobsen J, Visse R, Sørensen HP, Enghild JJ, Brew K, Wewer UM, Nagase H. Catalytic properties of ADAM12 and its domain deletion mutants. Biochemistry. 2008;**47**:537-547. DOI: 10.1021/bi701629c

[72] Fabunmi RP, Baker AH, Murray EJ, Booth RF, Newby AC. Divergent regulation by growth factors and cytokines of 95 kDa and 72 kDa gelatinases and tissue inhibitors or

metalloproteinases-1, -2, and -3 in rabbit aortic smooth muscle cells. The Biochemical Journal. 1996;**315**:335-342

[73] Overall CM. Regulation of tissue inhibitor of matrix metalloproteinase expression. Annals of the New York Academy of Sciences. 1994;**732**:51-64. DOI: 10.1111/j.1749-6632.1994.tb24724.x

[74] Hayakawa T, Yamashita K, Tanzawa K, Uchijima E, Iwata K. Growth-promoting activity of tissue inhibitor of metalloproteinases-1 (TIMP-1) for a wide range of cells. A possible new growth factor in serum. FEBS Letters. 1992;**298**:29-32. DOI: 10.1016/0014-5793(92)80015-9

[75] Hayakawa T, Yamashita K, Ohuchi E, Shinagawa A. Cell growth-promoting activity of tissue inhibitor of metalloproteinases-2 (TIMP-2). Journal of Cell Science. 1994;**107**:2373-2379

[76] Guedez L, Courtemanch L, Stetler-Stevenson M. Tissue inhibitor of metalloproteinase (TIMP)-1 induces differentiation and an antiapoptotic phenotype in germinal center B cells. Blood. 1998;**92**:1342-1349

[77] Valente P, Fassina G, Melchiori A, Masiello L, Cilli M, Vacca A, Onisto M, Santi L, Stetler-Stevenson WG, Albini A. TIMP-2 over-expression reduces invasion and angiogenesis and protects B16F10 melanoma cells from apoptosis. International Journal of Cancer. 1998;**75**:246-253. DOI: 10.1002/(SICI)1097-0215(19980119)75:2<246::AID-IJC13>3.0.CO;2-B

[78] Ahonen M, Poukkula M, Baker AH, Kashiwagi M, Nagase H, Eriksson JE, Kähäri VM. Tissue inhibitor of metalloproteinases-3 induces apoptosis in melanoma cells by stabilization of death receptors. Oncogene. 2003;**22**:2121-2134. DOI: 10.1038/sj.onc.1206292

[79] Murphy AN, Unsworth EJ, Stetler-Stevenson WG. Tissue inhibitor of metalloproteinases-2 inhibits bFGF-induced human microvascular endothelial cell proliferation. Journal of Cellular Physiology. 1993;**157**:351-358. DOI: 10.1002/jcp.1041570219

[80] Borth W. Alpha 2-macroglobulin, a multifunctional binding protein with targeting characteristics. The FASEB Journal. 1992;**6**:3345-3353

[81] Higashi S, Miyazaki K. Novel processing of beta-amyloid precursor protein catalyzed by membrane type 1 matrix metalloproteinase releases a fragment lacking the inhibitor domain against gelatinase A. Biochemistry. 2003;**42**:6514-6526. DOI: 10.1021/bi020643m

[82] Oh J, Takahashi R, Kondo S, Mizoguchi A, Adachi E, Sasahara RM, Nishimura S, Imamura Y, Kitayama H, Alexander DB, Ide C, Horan TP, Arakawa T, Yoshida H, Nishikawa S, Itoh Y, Seiki M, Itohara S, Takahashi C, Noda M. The membrane-anchored MMP inhibitor RECK is a key regulator of extracellular matrix integrity and angiogenesis. Cell. 2001;**107**:789-800. DOI: 10.1016/S0092-8674(01)00597-9

[83] Sledge GW Jr, Qulali M, Goulet R, Bone EA, Fife R. Effect of matrix metalloproteinase inhibitor batimastat on breast cancer regrowth and metastasis in athymic mice. Journal of the National Cancer Institute. 1995;**87**:1546-1450

[84] Low JA, Johnson MD, Bone EA, Dickson RB. The matrix metalloproteinase inhibitor batimastat (BB-94) retards human breast cancer solid tumor growth but not ascites formation in nude mice. Clinical Cancer Research. 1996;**2**:1207-1214

[85] Watson SA, Morris TM, Robinson G, Crimmin MJ, Brown PD, Hardcastle JD. Inhibition of organ invasion by the matrix metalloproteinase inhibitor batimastat (BB-94) in two human colon carcinoma metastasis models. Cancer Research. 1995;**55**:3629-3633

[86] Rao BG. Recent developments in the design of specific matrix metalloproteinase inhibitors aided by structural and computational studies. Current Pharmaceutical Design. 2005;**11**:295-322

[87] Mannello F, Tonti G, Papa S. Matrix metalloproteinase inhibitors as anticancer therapeutics. Current Cancer Drug Targets. 2005;**5**:285-298

[88] Sorsa T, Tjäderhane L, Konttinen YT, Lauhio A, Salo T, Lee HM, Golub LM, Brown DL, Mäntylä P. Matrix metalloproteinases: Contribution to pathogenesis, diagnosis and treatment of periodontal inflammation. Annals of Medicine. 2006;**38**:306-321. DOI: 10.1080/07853890600800103

[89] Overall CM, Kleifeld O. Toward third generation matrix metalloproteinase inhibitors for cancer therapy. British Journal of Cancer. 2006;**94**:941-946. DOI: 10.1038/sj.bjc.6603043

[90] Shiryaev SA, Remacle AG, Golubkov VS, Ingvarsen S, Porse A, Behrendt N, Cieplak P, Strongin AY. A monoclonal antibody interferes with TIMP-2 binding and incapacitates the MMP-2-activating function of multifunctional, pro-tumorigenic MMP-14/MT1-MMP. Oncogene. 2013;**2**:e80. DOI: 10.1038/oncsis.2013.44

[91] Murphy G. Tissue inhibitors of metalloproteinases. Genome Biology. 2011;**12**:233. DOI: 10.1186/gb-2011-12-11-233

[92] Vandenbroucke RE, Libert C. Is there new hope for therapeutic matrix metalloproteinase inhibition? Nature Reviews. Drug Discovery. 2014;**13**:904-927. DOI: 10.1038/nrd4390

[93] Shiomi T, Lemaitre V, D'Armiento J, Okada Y. Matrix metalloproteinases, a disintegrin and metalloproteinases, and a disintegrin and metalloproteinases with thrombospondin motifs in non-neoplastic diseases. Pathology International. 2010;**60**:477-496. DOI: 10.1111/j.1440-1827.2010.02547.x

[94] Ye S, Eriksson P, Hamsten A, Kurkinen M, Humphries SE, Henney AM. Progression of coronary atherosclerosis is associated with a common genetic variant of the human stromelysin-1 promoter which results in reduced gene expression. The Journal of Biological Chemistry. 1996;**271**:13055-13060

[95] Zhang B, Ye S, Herrmann SM, Eriksson P, de Maat M, Evans A, et al. Functional polymorphism in the regulatory region of gelatinase B gene in relation to severity of coronary atherosclerosis. Circulation. 1999;**99**:1788-1794

[96] Zhu C, Odeberg J, Hamsten A, Eriksson P. Allele-specific MMP-3 transcription under in vivo conditions. Biochemical and Biophysical Research Communications. 2006;**348**:1150-1156. DOI: 10.1016/j.bbrc.2006.07.174

[97] Ye S, Watts GF, Mandalia S, Humphries SE, Henney AM. Preliminary report: Genetic variation in the human stromelysin promoter is associated with progression of coronary atherosclerosis. British Heart Journal. 1995;**73**:209-215

[98] Humphries SE, Luong LA, Talmud PJ, Frick MH, Kesaniemi YA, Pasternack A, et al. The 5A/6A polymorphism in the promoter of the stromelysin-1 (MMP-3) gene predicts progression of angiographically determined coronary artery disease in men in the LOCAT gemfibrozil study. Lopid coronary angiography trial. Atherosclerosis. 1998;**139**:49-56

[99] Hirashiki A, Yamada Y, Murase Y, Suzuki Y, Kataoka H, Morimoto Y, et al. Association of gene polymorphisms with coronary artery disease in low- or high-risk subjects defined by conventional risk factors. Journal of the American College of Cardiology. 2003;**42**:1429-1437

[100] Beyzade S, Zhang S, Wong YK, Day IN, Eriksson P, Ye S. Influences of matrix metalloproteinase-3 gene variation on extent of coronary atherosclerosis and risk of myocardial infarction. Journal of the American College of Cardiology. 2003;**41**:2130-2137

[101] Schwarz A, Haberbosch W, Tillmanns H, Gardemann A. The stromelysin-1 5A/6A promoter polymorphism is a disease marker for the extent of coronary heart disease. Disease Markers. 2002;**18**:121-128

[102] Ye S, Gale CR, Martyn CN. Variation in the matrix metalloproteinase-1 gene and risk of coronary heart disease. European Heart Journal. 2003;**24**:1668-1671

[103] Ghilardi G, Biondi ML, DeMonti M, Turri O, Guagnellini E, Scorza R. Matrix metalloproteinase-1 and matrix metalloproteinase-3 gene promoter polymorphisms are associated with carotid artery stenosis. Stroke. 2002;**33**:2408-2412

[104] Rauramaa R, Vaisanen SB, Luong LA, Schmidt-Trucksass A, Penttila IM, Bouchard C, et al. Stromelysin-1 and interleukin-6 gene promoter polymorphisms are determinants of asymptomatic carotid artery atherosclerosis. Arteriosclerosis, Thrombosis, and Vascular Biology. 2000;**20**:2657-2662

[105] Rundek T, Elkind MS, Pittman J, Boden-Albala B, Martin S, Humphries SE, et al. Carotid intima-media thickness is associated with allelic variants of stromelysin-1, interleukin-6, and hepatic lipase genes: The Northern Manhattan prospective cohort study. Stroke. 2002;**33**:1420-1423

[106] Djuric T, Zivkovic M, Radak D, Jekic D, Radak S, Stojkovic L, et al. Association of MMP-3 5A/6A gene polymorphism with susceptibility to carotid atherosclerosis. Clinical Biochemistry. 2008;**41**:1326-1329. DOI: 10.1016/j.clinbiochem.2008.08.081

[107] Beilby JP, Chapman CM, Palmer LJ, McQuillan BM, Thompson PL, Hung J. Stromelysin-1 (MMP-3) gene 5A/6A promoter polymorphism is associated with blood pressure in a community population. Journal of Hypertension. 2005;**23**:537-542

[108] Medley TL, Kingwell BA, Gatzka CD, Pillay P, Cole TJ. Matrix metalloproteinase-3 genotype contributes to age-related aortic stiffening through modulation of gene and protein expression. Circulation Research. 2003;**92**:1254-1261. DOI: 10.1161/01.res.0000076891.24317.ca

[109] Zivkovic M, Djuric T, Alavantic D, Mecanin S, Stankovic A. Association of ACE I/D and MMP-3 5A/6A gene polymorphisms with hypertension in Serbian males. Archives of Biological Sciences. 2006;**58**:205-210

[110] Terashima M, Akita H, Kanazawa K, Inoue N, Yamada S, Ito K, et al. Stromelysin promoter 5A/6A polymorphism is associated with acute myocardial infarction. Circulation. 1999;**99**:2717-2719

[111] Nojiri T, Morita H, Imai Y, Maemura K, Ohno M, Ogasawara K, et al. Genetic variations of matrix metalloproteinase-1 and -3 promoter regions and their associations with susceptibility to myocardial infarction in Japanese. International Journal of Cardiology. 2003;**92**:181-186

[112] Pollanen PJ, Lehtimaki T, Mikkelsson J, Ilveskoski E, Kunnas T, Perola M, et al. Matrix metalloproteinase3 and 9 gene promoter polymorphisms: Joint action of two loci as a risk factor for coronary artery complicated plaques. Atherosclerosis. 2005;**180**:73-78. DOI: 10.1016/j.atherosclerosis.2004.10.041

[113] Abilleira S, Bevan S, Markus HS. The role of genetic variants of matrix metalloproteinases in coronary and carotid atherosclerosis. Journal of Medical Genetics. 2006;**43**:897-901. DOI: 10.1136/jmg.2006.040808

[114] Koch W, de Waha A, Hoppmann P, Schomig A, Kastrati A. Haplotypes and 5A/6A polymorphism of the matrix metalloproteinase-3 gene in coronary disease: Case–control study and a meta-analysis. Atherosclerosis. 2010;**208**:171-176. DOI: 10.1016/j.atherosclerosis.2009.08.021

[115] Morris DR, Biros E, Cronin O, Kuivaniemi H, Golledge J. The association of genetic variants of matrix metalloproteinases with abdominal aortic aneurysm: A systematic review and meta-analysis. Heart. 2014;**100**:295-302. DOI: 10.1136/heartjnl-2013-304129

[116] Saratzis A, Bown MJ, Wild B, Nightingale P, Smith J, Johnson C, et al. Association between seven single nucleotide polymorphisms involved in inflammation and proteolysis and abdominal aortic aneurysm. Journal of Vascular Surgery. 2015;**61**:1120-1128 e1121. DOI: 10.1016/j.jvs.2013.11.099

[117] Newby AC, Zaltsman AB. Fibrous cap formation or destruction--the critical importance of vascular smooth muscle cell proliferation, migration and matrix formation. Cardiovascular Research. 1999;**41**:345-360

[118] Zhang B, Henney A, Eriksson P, Hamsten A, Watkins H, Ye S. Genetic variation at the matrix metalloproteinase-9 locus on chromosome 20q12.2-13.1. Human Genetics. 1999;**105**:418-423

[119] Maqbool A, Turner NA, Galloway S, Riches K, O'Regan DJ, Porter KE. The -1562C/T MMP-9 promoter polymorphism does not predict MMP-9 expression levels or invasive capacity in saphenous vein smooth muscle cells cultured from different patients. Atherosclerosis. 2009;**207**:458-465. DOI: 10.1016/j.atherosclerosis.2009.05.028

[120] Morgan AR, Zhang B, Tapper W, Collins A, Ye S. Haplotypic analysis of the MMP-9 gene in relation to coronary artery disease. Journal of Molecular Medicine (Berlin). 2003;**81**:321-326. DOI: 10.1007/s00109-003-0441-z

[121] Cho HJ, Chae IH, Park KW, Ju JR, Oh S, Lee MM, et al. Functional polymorphism in the promoter region of the gelatinase B gene in relation to coronary artery disease and restenosis after percutaneous coronary intervention. Journal of Human Genetics. 2002;**47**:88-91. DOI: 10.1007/s100380200006

[122] Wang J, Warzecha D, Wilcken D, Wang XL. Polymorphism in the gelatinase B gene and the severity of coronary arterial stenosis. Clinical Science (London, England). 2001;**101**:87-92

[123] Haberbosch W, Gardemann A. Gelatinase B C(−1562)T polymorphism in relation to ischaemic heart disease. Scandinavian Journal of Clinical and Laboratory Investigation. 2005;**65**:513-522. DOI: 10.1080/00365510500206575

[124] Niu W, Qi Y. Matrix metalloproteinase family gene polymorphisms and risk for coronary artery disease: Systematic review and meta-analysis. Heart. 2012;**98**:1483-1491. DOI: 10.1136/heartjnl-2012-302085

[125] Horne BD, Camp NJ, Carlquist JF, Muhlestein JB, Kolek MJ, Nicholas ZP, et al. Multiple-polymorphism associations of 7 matrix metalloproteinase and tissue inhibitor metalloproteinase genes with myocardial infarction and angiographic coronary artery disease. American Heart Journal. 2007;**154**:751-758. DOI: 10.1016/j.ahj.2007.06.030

[126] Yasmin, McEniery CM, O'Shaughnessy KM, Harnett P, Arshad A, Wallace S, et al. Variation in the human matrix metalloproteinase-9 gene is associated with arterial stiffness in healthy individuals. Arteriosclerosis, Thrombosis, and Vascular Biology. 2006;**26**:1799-1805. DOI: 10.1161/01.atv.0000227717.46157.32

[127] Opstad TB, Pettersen AA, Weiss TW, Akra S, Ovstebo R, Arnesen H, et al. Genetic variation, gene-expression and circulating levels of matrix metalloproteinase-9 in patients with stable coronary artery disease. Clinica Chimica Acta. 2012;**413**:113-120. DOI: 10.1016/j.cca.2011.09.004

[128] Mishra A, Srivastava A, Mittal T, Garg N, Mittal B. Association of matrix metalloproteinases (MMP2, MMP7 and MMP9) genetic variants with left ventricular dysfunction in coronary artery disease patients. Clinica Chimica Acta. 2012;**413**:1668-1674. DOI: 10.1016/j.cca.2012.05.012

[129] Duellman T, Warren CL, Peissig P, Wynn M, Yang J. Matrix metalloproteinase-9 genotype as a potential genetic marker for abdominal aortic aneurysm. Circulation. Cardiovascular Genetics. 2012;**5**:529-537. DOI: 10.1161/circgenetics.112.963082

[130] Yuan M, Zhan Q, Duan X, Song B, Zeng S, Chen X, et al. A functional polymorphism at miR-491-5p binding site in the 3′-UTR of MMP-9 gene confers increased risk for atherosclerotic cerebral infarction in a Chinese population. Atherosclerosis. 2013;**226**:447-452. DOI: 10.1016/j.atherosclerosis.2012.11.026

[131] Price SJ, Greaves DR, Watkins H. Identification of novel, functional genetic variants in the human matrix metalloproteinase-2 gene: Role of Sp1 in allele-specific transcriptional regulation. The Journal of Biological Chemistry. 2001;**276**:7549-7558. DOI: 10.1074/jbc.M010242200

[132] Vasku A, Goldbergova M, Izakovicova Holla L, Siskova L, Groch L, Beranek M, et al. A haplotype constituted of four MMP-2 promoter polymorphisms (−1575G/a, −1306C/T, −790 T/G and −735C/T) is associated with coronary triple-vessel disease. Matrix Biology. 2004;**22**:585-591. DOI: 10.1016/j.matbio.2003.10.004

[133] Rutter JL, Mitchell TI, Buttice G, Meyers J, Gusella JF, Ozelius LJ, et al. A single nucleotide polymorphism in the matrix metalloproteinase-1 promoter creates an Ets binding site and augments transcription. Cancer Research. 1998;**58**:5321-5325

[134] Pearce E, Tregouet DA, Samnegard A, Morgan AR, Cox C, Hamsten A, et al. Haplotype effect of the matrix metalloproteinase-1 gene on risk of myocardial infarction. Circulation Research. 2005;**97**:1070-1076. DOI: 10.1161/01.res.0000189302.03303.11

[135] Hlatky MA, Ashley E, Quertermous T, Boothroyd DB, Ridker P, Southwick A, et al. Matrix metalloproteinase circulating levels, genetic polymorphisms, and susceptibility to acute myocardial infarction among patients with coronary artery disease. American Heart Journal. 2007;**154**:1043-1051. DOI: 10.1016/j.ahj.2007.06.042

[136] Cheng YC, Kao WH, Mitchell BD, O'Connell JR, Shen H, McArdle PF, et al. Genome-wide association scan identifies variants near matrix metalloproteinase (MMP) genes on chromosome 11q21-22 strongly associated with serum MMP-1 levels. Circulation. Cardiovascular Genetics. 2009;**2**:329-337. DOI: 10.1161/circgenetics.108.834986

[137] Wang H, Parry S, Macones G, Sammel MD, Ferrand PE, Kuivaniemi H, et al. Functionally significant SNP MMP8 promoter haplotypes and preterm premature rupture of membranes (PPROM). Human Molecular Genetics. 2004;**13**:2659-2669. DOI: 10.1093/hmg/ddh287

[138] Laxton RC, Hu Y, Duchene J, Zhang F, Zhang Z, Leung KY, et al. A role of matrix metalloproteinase-8 in atherosclerosis. Circulation Research. 2009;**105**:921-929. DOI: 10.1161/circresaha.109.200279

[139] Djuric T, Stankovic A, Koncar I, Radak D, Davidovic L, Alavantic D, et al. Association of MMP-8 promoter gene polymorphisms with carotid atherosclerosis: Preliminary study. Atherosclerosis. 2011;**219**:673-678. DOI: 10.1016/j.atherosclerosis.2011.08.025

[140] Li C, Jin XP, Zhu M, Chen QL, Wang F, Hu XF, et al. Positive association of MMP 14 gene polymorphism with vulnerable carotid plaque formation in a Han Chinese population. Scandinavian Journal of Clinical and Laboratory Investigation. 2014;**74**:248-253. DOI: 10.3109/00365513.2013.879731

[141] Lehrke M, Greif M, Broedl UC, Lebherz C, Laubender RP, Becker A, et al. MMP-1 serum levels predict coronary atherosclerosis in humans. Cardiovascular Diabetology. 2009;**8**:50. DOI: 10.1186/1475-2840-8-50

[142] Blankenberg S, Rupprecht HJ, Poirier O, Bickel C, Smieja M, Hafner G, et al. Plasma concentrations and genetic variation of matrix metalloproteinase 9 and prognosis of patients with cardiovascular disease. Circulation. 2003;**107**:1579-1585. DOI: 10.1161/01.cir.0000058700.41738.12

[143] Jefferis BJ, Whincup P, Welsh P, Wannamethee G, Rumley A, Lennon L, et al. Prospective study of matrix metalloproteinase-9 and risk of myocardial infarction and stroke in older men and women. Atherosclerosis. 2010;**208**:557-563. DOI: 10.1016/j.atherosclerosis.2009.08.018

[144] Tuomainen AM, Nyyssonen K, Laukkanen JA, Tervahartiala T, Tuomainen TP, Salonen JT, et al. Serum matrix metalloproteinase-8 concentrations are associated with cardiovascular outcome in men. Arteriosclerosis, Thrombosis, and Vascular Biology. 2007;**27**:2722-2728. DOI: 10.1161/atvbaha.107.154831

[145] Hasty KA, Jeffrey JJ, Hibbs MS, Welgus HG. The collagen substrate specificity of human neutrophil collagenase. The Journal of Biological Chemistry. 1987;**262**:10048-10052

[146] Momiyama Y, Ohmori R, Tanaka N, Kato R, Taniguchi H, Adachi T, et al. High plasma levels of matrix metalloproteinase-8 in patients with unstable angina. Atherosclerosis. 2010;**209**:206-210. DOI: 10.1016/j.atherosclerosis.2009.07.037

[147] Djuric T, Zivkovic M, Stankovic A, Kolakovic A, Jekic D, Selakovic V, et al. Plasma levels of matrix metalloproteinase-8 in patients with carotid atherosclerosis. Journal of Clinical Laboratory Analysis. 2010;**24**:246-251. DOI: 10.1002/jcla.20393

[148] Fertin M, Lemesle G, Turkieh A, Beseme O, Chwastyniak M, Amouyel P, et al. Serum MMP-8: A novel indicator of left ventricular remodeling and cardiac outcome in patients after acute myocardial infarction. PLoS One. 2013;**8**:e71280. DOI: 10.1371/journal.pone.0071280

[149] Brkic M, Balusu S, Libert C, Vandenbroucke RE. Friends or foes: Matrix metalloproteinases and their multifaceted roles in neurodegenerative diseases. Mediators of Inflammation. 2015;**2015**:620581. DOI: 10.1155/2015/620581

[150] Nelissen I, Vandenbroeck K, Fiten P, Hillert J, Olsson T, Marrosu MG, et al. Polymorphism analysis suggests that the gelatinase B gene is not a susceptibility factor for multiple sclerosis. Journal of Neuroimmunology. 2000;**105**:58-63

[151] Benesova Y, Vasku A, Stourac P, Hladikova M, Beranek M, Kadanka Z, et al. Matrix metalloproteinase-9 and matrix metalloproteinase-2 gene polymorphisms in multiple sclerosis. Journal of Neuroimmunology. 2008;**205**:105-109. DOI: 10.1016/j.jneuroim.2008.08.007

[152] He X, Zhang L, Yao X, Hu J, Yu L, Jia H, et al. Association studies of MMP-9 in Parkinson's disease and amyotrophic lateral sclerosis. PLoS One. 2013;**8**:e73777. DOI: 10.1371/journal.pone.0073777

[153] La Russa A, Cittadella R, De Marco EV, Valentino P, Andreoli V, Trecroci F, et al. Single nucleotide polymorphism in the MMP-9 gene is associated with susceptibility to develop multiple sclerosis in an Italian case–control study. Journal of Neuroimmunology. 2010;**225**:175-179. DOI: 10.1016/j.jneuroim.2010.04.016

[154] Fernandes KS, Brum DG, Sandrim VC, Guerreiro CT, Barreira AA, Tanus-Santos JE. Matrix metalloproteinase-9 genotypes and haplotypes are associated with multiple sclerosis and with the degree of disability of the disease. Journal of Neuroimmunology. 2009;**214**:128-131. DOI: 10.1016/j.jneuroim.2009.07.004

[155] Djuric T, Zivkovic M, Stankovic A, Dincic E, Raicevic R, Alavantic D. Association of the MMP-3 5A/6A gene polymorphism with multiple sclerosis in patients from Serbia. Journal of the Neurological Sciences. 2008;**267**:62-65. DOI: 10.1016/j.jns.2007.09.037

[156] Gasparovic I, Cizmarevic NS, Lovrecic L, Perkovic O, Lavtar P, Sepcic J, et al. MMP-2 -1575G/A polymorphism modifies the onset of optic neuritis as a first presenting symptom in MS? Journal of Neuroimmunology. 2015;**286**:13-15. DOI: 10.1016/j.jneuroim.2015.06.014

[157] Reitz C, van Rooij FJ, Soares HD, de Maat MP, Hofman A, Witteman JC, et al. Matrix metalloproteinase 3 haplotypes and plasma amyloid beta levels: The Rotterdam study. Neurobiology of Aging. 2010;**31**:715-718. DOI: 10.1016/j.neurobiolaging.2008.05.033

[158] Reitz C, van Rooij FJ, de Maat MP, den Heijer T, Hofman A, Witteman JC, et al. Matrix metalloproteinase 3 haplotypes and dementia and Alzheimer's disease. The Rotterdam Study. Neurobiol Aging. 2008;**29**:874-881. DOI: 10.1016/j.neurobiolaging.2007.01.001

Section 2

Involvement of Matrix Metalloproteinases in Cardiovascular Diseases

Chapter 2

Heart Remodelation: Role of MMPs

Marek Pytliak, Viliam Vaník and Peter Bojčík

Additional information is available at the end of the chapter

http://dx.doi.org/10.5772/intechopen.71662

Abstract

Myocardium is comprised of a number of cell types. Although most plentiful by volume, cardiac myocytes are greatly outnumbered by nonmyocyte cells, the latter constituting approximately 70% of all myocardial cells, of which approximately 90% are cardiac fibroblasts (CFBs). To maintain the integrity of the cardiac extracellular matrix (ECM) is one of the primary functions of cardiac fibroblasts. ECM represents a network structure that provides the structural and functional integrity to the heart. Besides that, it also contains a high number of cytokines and growth factors with effects on cardiac function and cardiac cells. Cardiac ECM also mediates the mechanical connection between the cardiomyocytes, CFBs, and blood. In addition to producing ECM proteins, CFBs also produce ECM-regulatory proteins – matrix metalloproteinases (MMPs), which can degrade ECM proteins – and their inhibitors, tissue inhibitors of metalloproteinases (TIMPs). To date, 26 MMPs have been cloned and characterized in vertebrates. From these, MMP1, MMP3, MMP8, MMP13, MMP2, MMP9, MMP12, MMP28, and the membrane-type MMPs (MT1-MMP/MMP14) have been identified to be involved in the myocardial remodeling. The role of higher MMPs in the cardiovascular system is less well explored.

Keywords: MMPs, heart remodeling, heart failure, acute coronary syndrome, atherosclerosis

1. Introduction

The heart is a muscular pump composed of cardiac myocytes and interstitial components. Although most plentiful by volume, cardiac myocytes are greatly outnumbered by nonmyocyte cells, the latter constituting approximately 70% of all myocardial cells, of which approximately 90% are cardiac fibroblasts (CFBs) [1]. Whereas cardiac myocytes and the coronary vasculature are central to the contractile function and viability of the myocardium, so too is the extracellular matrix, or cardiac interstitium serve as supporting structure. Collagen fibers, the major structural proteins of the interstitium, serve several functions showed in **Table 1** [2].

Scaffold supporting muscle cells and blood vessels
Lateral connections between cells and muscle bundles to govern architecture
Acting as a signal transducer for cell-cell communication modulating cell motility, survival, and cell proliferation
Coordinating the delivery of force, generated by myocytes, to the ventricular chamber
Determinants of diastolic and systolic myocardial stiffness
Serving to resist myocardial deformation and maintaining shape and wall thickness

Table 1. Functions of the collagen matrix in the heart.

The ECM is crucial to maintain appropriate cardiac integrity and pump function. Conversely, disruption of ECM homeostasis is a central factor for cardiac dysfunction, pathologic remodeling, and fibrosis following cardiac injury.

Most myocardial collagen fibers consist of collagen types I and III, which (depending on species) account for approximately 80% and 10% of collagen in the healthy heart, respectively. The nonstructural compartment of the ECM houses a variety of proteins, which are vital for ECM plasticity, and can be divided into three major groups: glycoproteins, proteoglycans, and glycosaminoglycans [3].

In addition to a fibrillar collagen network, a basement membrane, proteoglycans, and glycosaminoglycans, the myocardial ECM contains a large reservoir of bioactive molecules. For example, the concentration of angiotensin II (ANG II) and endothelin (ET)-1 is over 100-fold higher within the myocardial interstitium than in plasma. ECM also acts as a reservoir for growth factors (such as transforming growth factor-β), which are stored within the myocardial interstitium in a latent form and directly influence myocardial ECM synthesis and degradation. Moreover, mechanical stimuli such as stress or strain are transduced through the myocardial ECM to the cardiac myocyte, which in turn would directly affect myocyte growth and ECM remodelation [4, 5].

2. Normal heart interstitium

2.1. Collagens

As mentioned above, collagen is the predominant structural component of the ECM. It has been classified into three components:

1. epimysium – the collagenous matrix that lies below the endothelium of the epicardium and endocardium and surrounding the entire muscle
2. endomysium – endomysial collagen fibers consist of fibrils that connect adjoining myocytes to one another and to their neighboring capillaries
3. perimysium – surrounding and interconnecting groups of myocytes. It consists of tendon-like extensions of the epimysium that arborize into a weave to aggregate myocytes into myofibers [6].

http://dx.doi.org/10.5772/intechopen.71662

Collagen synthesis and degradation in the healthy heart is an ongoing balanced process. The major types of collagen present in the myocardium of the left ventricle are I and III, with type I predominating. Type I collagen is the most abundant collagen of the human body, which forms large, eosinophilic fibers known as collagen fibers. The COL1A1 gene produces the pro-alpha1 (I) chain, and pro-alpha2 (I) chain is produced by the COL1A2 gene. Two chains of pro-alpha1 (I) combine together with one pro-alpha2 (I) chain to make a molecule of type I procollagen. These molecules must be processed by enzymes outside the cell. After that, they arrange themselves into long, thin fibrils that cross-link to one another in the spaces around cells, which leads to the formation of very strong fibers of the mature type I collagen. In humans, collagen alpha-1 (III) chain is encoded by the COL3A1 gene located on chromosome 2. Collagen alpha-1 (III) chain is a precursor for collagen III that is found in extensible connective tissues [7, 8].

Myocytes are surrounded by a basement membrane (BM). The principal structural component of the basement membrane is collagen type IV, while collagens I and III are arranged in sequential layers of organization of the BM. However, collagen does not only fulfill the architectural function. It is also involved in intracellular signal transduction. Via a β1 integrin-dependent mechanism, collagen can inhibit apoptosis and so promotes cell survival in vitro. Collagen is also implicated in the induction of proliferation via FAK activation and downstream signaling pathways (Src, MEK, PI3-kinase, and p38 MAPK). In addition, collagen participates in cell spreading through p130Cas phosphorylation via FAK-dependent and FAK-independent integrin receptor pathways [9, 10]. Finally, collagen plays a key role in cell migration through the activation of FAK and PI3-K, leading to elevated Rac1 activity as a downstream consequence in activated cell migration [11].

2.2. Cardiac fibroblasts

Cardiac myocytes occupy approximately 75% of normal myocardial tissue volume, but they account for only 30–40% of cell numbers. Cardiac fibroblasts (CFBs) have the highest cell population in the myocardium, accounting for about two-thirds of the cells.

Fibroblasts (FBs) are present in every tissue in the body [5]. They are of mesenchymal origin and are morphologically flat and spindle-shaped, with multiple processes. CFBs in the myocardium lack a basement membrane, which distinguishes them from all other cells. In the past, FBs have been considered for a homogeneous cell population. Over time, though, it has become clear that FBs from various tissues have different properties and functions. Fibroblasts are found throughout the cardiac tissue, surrounding myocytes and bridging "spaces" between myocardial tissue layers, so that, in essence, every cardiomyocyte is closely related to a fibroblast in normal cardiac tissue. The primary function of FBs is to produce structural proteins that form the extracellular matrix. Under physiological circumstances, this is a constructive process. On the other site, hyperactivity of cardiac fibroblasts can result in excess production and deposition of ECM proteins that can lead to fibrosis. Fibrosis of the myocardium affects the cardiac structure and function in the negative way. Fibroblasts also produce a number of cytokines, peptides, and enzymes including matrix metalloproteinases (MMPs) and their inhibitors, tissue inhibitors of metalloproteinases (TIMPs) that directly affect the ECM turnover and homeostasis. In turn, as a feedback, function of fibroblasts can also be regulated by MMPs and TIMPs [12, 13].

CFBs can differentiate into myofibroblasts (myoFBs), more mobile and contractile elements with a greater synthetic potential to produce ECM proteins. Incentives for this differentiation are various stimuli, most commonly myocardial injury. MyoFBs were identified by Gabbiani in 1971 [14]. They only appear after cardiac injury and are not found in healthy myocardium. Cardiac myoFBs, similar to CFBs, are nonexcitable cells, which express a number of smooth muscle cell markers, such as alpha smooth muscle actin (αSMA), smooth muscle myosin heavy chain, paxillin, vinculin, and tensin, that are not typically expressed in quiescent CFBs [15].

2.3. Matrix metalloproteinases in the normal heart

MMPs are a family of more than 25 species of zinc-dependent proteases that are synthesized as inactive zymogens (pro-MMPs). They are essential for normal tissue remodeling in processes such as bone growth, wound healing, and reproduction. Moreover, increased induction and elaboration of MMPs have been identified to hold biological significance in a number of pathological conditions that include cancer, inflammatory disease, and cardiovascular disease. MMPs are the predominant proteases responsible for degradation of the ECM proteins. To date, 26 MMPs have been cloned and characterized in vertebrates. From these, MMP1, MMP3, MMP8, MMP13, MMP2, MMP9, MMP12, MMP28, and the membrane-type MMPs (MT1-MMP/MMP14) have been identified to be involved in the myocardial remodeling. The role of higher MMPs in the cardiovascular system is less well explored [16].

The interstitial collagenase (MMP-1), neutrophil collagenase (MMP-8), and collagenase-3 (MMP-13) possess high substrate specificity for fibrillar collagens, as well as other ECM proteins such as aggrecan, perlican, versican, and proteoglycans. The important substrates for MMP-1 and MMP-13 within the myocardium include the fibrillar collagens such as collagen type I and III [17].

The gelatinases (MMP-2 and MMP-9) demonstrate substrate affinity for denatured fibrillar collagen, basement membrane proteins such as collagen type IV, fibronectin, and laminin. MMP-2 and MMP-9 also exhibit proteolytic activity against elastin and proteoglycans. Past studies have demonstrated that MMP-9 is synthesized by myocytes, fibroblasts, and smooth muscle cells. Moreover, neutrophils have also been reported to be a potential source of MMP-9 [18].

Stromelysin (MMP-3) degrades all basement membrane proteins, elastin, and proteoglycans.

MMP-7 lacks the hemopexin domain, which seems to be critical in substrate recognition. Therefore, MMP-7 has a wide substrate portfolio and possesses proteolytic activity against the fibrillar collagens I and III, basement membrane proteins (collagen IV and fibronectin), and proteoglycans [19].

MMP-12 (macrophage elastase) has broad substrate specificity for extracellular components and is shown to be a key player in tissue remodeling associated with many pathological conditions such as chronic inflammation and fibrosis [20].

During ECM degradation (in physiological ECM turnover or pathological ECM remodeling), collagen fibers are degraded into smaller peptides. After that, telopeptides in the N-terminals or C-terminals of collagen molecules are cleaved. The propeptide from the carboxy-terminal or the amino-terminal propeptides of collagen type I (PICP, PINP) and both terminals of collagen type III (PIIICP, PIIINP) that uprise during biosynthesis of these collagens can be considered as biomarkers of collagen synthesis, as they are released in a stoichiometric manner. Similarly, the C-terminal or N-terminal telopeptides of collagen type I (CITP, NITP) and type III (CIIITP, NIIITP), produced by degradation of these collagens, are considered biomarkers of collagen degradation [21].

3. MMPs in heart disease

Matrix metalloproteinases and their inhibitors have a fundamental role in the remodeling of the ECM in both normal and pathological conditions. In addition, MMPs have an important role in cardiovascular diseases, including acute and chronic heart failure (CHF), acute myocardial infarction, atherosclerosis, and cardiomyopathies.

3.1. MMPs in acute heart failure

Although the relationship between MMPs and chronic heart failure (CHF) has been well investigated, we have poor information about changes in the serum levels of MMPs in patients with acute heart failure (AHF). In patients with AHF, production of MMPs is affected by several mechanisms including changes in hemodynamic conditions and neurohormonal and inflammatory factors. Biolo et al. reported that some markers of extracellular matrix turnover (MMP-2, TIMP-1, and procollagen type III N-terminal peptide) were elevated in patients with AHF syndrome. The increase in ECM turnover may be associated with an acceleration of pathological remodeling. The decrease in the concentrations of MMP-2 during the acute phase of heart failure may represent the deceleration of myocardial remodeling and maybe a better prognosis of AHF [22]. In the study of Shirakabe et al., the serum levels of MMP-2 were measured on 83 AHF patients before starting treatment (day 1), on day 3 and day 7 after admission to the hospital, and before discharge. They found rapid and significant decrease in the MMP-2 concentrations on day 3 compared to day 1, whereas the MMP-2 levels were not significantly different on day 7 and at predischarge. Authors also evaluated the relationship between ΔMMP-2 (defined as the changes in MMP-2 concentrations from day 1 to day 3) and HF events including cardiac death, readmission to hospital for HF, and controllable HF. The levels of MMP-2 were significantly ($p = 0.004$) more decreased in the event-free group compared to the group with events mentioned above. The results of multivariate logistic regression model for predicting HF events found that the specific factor for HF events was ΔMMP-2. Rapid decrease in MMP-2 concentration after acute heart failure event thus may be important for better clinical outcome in patients with AHF [23].

Hadipurnomo et al. examined samples of 122 consecutive patients with acute coronary syndrome (ACS) treated in ICCU of which 47 showed the signs of AHF. The level of MMP-9 was examined a time at admission in ICCU, before thrombolysis was done. The acute heart failure accompanying ACS had Killip II-IV scores. The level of MMP-9 in ACS with AHF was significantly higher than in ACS without AHF, with p value <0.001 [24]. Similar results were presented in a study of Jong et al. who investigated the serum concentrations and activities of MMP-9 in patients with heart failure developed after AMI. Twenty-eight patients post-AMI and without heart failure (Killip I, cardiopulmonary compensated) and twenty-seven post-AMI patients who developed heart failure (Killip II-III, decompensated) were selected to evaluate the serum levels and activities of MMP-9. It was observed that both serum levels and activities of MMP-9 significantly increased ($P < 0.01$) in decompensated group compared to compensated group. The highly elevated serum MMP-9 concentration of decompensated patients was not related to inflammatory or localized infarct area of myocardium. Authors suggest that the increase of MMP-9 levels and activity may be used as a new marker to diagnose the development of heart failure in patients post-MI [25]. Levosimendan is calcium sensitizer, cardiotonic agent that binds to troponin C with high affinity. This pharmaceutical agent promotes cardiac contractility without increasing myocardial oxygen demand. Tziakas, et al. demonstrated that levosimendan significantly reduced MMP-2 levels in patients with acute decompensation of chronic heart failure [26].

3.2. MMPs in the chronic heart failure

Essential points in the development and progression of HF include changes in the structure, composition, and geometry of the left ventricular (LV) myocardium, which has been generically termed LV remodeling. Left ventricular remodeling that precedes and occurs along the development of HF is strongly associated with adverse clinical outcomes in HF patients with systolic dysfunction. Changes in the overall structure and function of extracellular matrix directly contribute to the adverse LV remodeling. There are fairly distinct patterns of LV remodeling that occur and are dependent on the initial pathophysiological stimulus but, once instigated, LV remodeling is an important predictor for the development and progression of HF. The activity of MMPs has been shown to be increased in the progression of heart failure. The level of MMPs and their induction and activation systems are increased in pathological specimens of human heart failure.

As mentioned above, sources of MMPs in the heart are fibroblasts, myocytes, endothelial cells, and inflammatory cells, e.g. monocytes that infiltrate the myocardium in several circumstances. In heart failure, plasma levels of tumor necrosis factor-α (TNF-α) are increased. Monocytes stimulated by TNF-α are capable to produce MMP-9. It is supposed that monocytes and other blood elements may serve as carriers of MMP-9, which is synthesized before they infiltrate the myocardium. Observation that in reperfusion of myocardium after acute infarction, infiltrating neutrophils are the predominant source of MMP-9 and activating enzymes supports this hypothesis.

Cyclic strain has been shown to induce a number of MMPs, such as the gelatinase MMP-2. In myocardial biopsies performed in patients with LV pressure overload secondary to aortic stenosis, increased MMP-2 expression and activity were identified. In patients with LV hypertrophy and HF with a history of hypertension, plasma levels of MMP-2 were significantly increased compared with age-matched control subjects. For example, in the study of Spinale et al., left ventricular myocardial MMP activity (measured by zymography) increased by >2-fold in nonischemic dilated cardiomyopathy (DCM) and ischemic DCM when compared with MMP activity in normal hearts. Abundant concentration of MMP-9 was observed in both forms of DCM. MMP-2 and MMP-3 activities were increased with nonischemic DCM. On the other site, MMP-1 levels were decreased in both forms of DCM [27].

In patients with CHF, elevated serum levels of MMP-1 and TIMP-1 have been observed. This finding indicates a predominance of collagenolytic activity, which results in an increase of serum concentrations of CITP (type I collagen carboxy-terminal telopeptide), a marker of collagen degradation. A report from López et al. shows an increase of the MMP-1/TIMP-1 ratio (both in tissue and serum samples) in hypertensive systolic heart failure compared with hypertensive diastolic heart failure [28]. On the other hand, some other studies analyzed human myocardium from explanted hearts from patients undergoing heart transplantation. They have found decreased MMP-1 expression and notable increase in TIMP-1 concentration [29]. Finally, study of George et al. found that MMP-2 but not TIMP-1 is an independent predictor of mortality in patients with CHF [30]. In the study of Jordán et al., patients with CHF had lower levels of MMP-1 and higher levels of TIMP-1 and TIMP-1/MMP-1 ratio than controls. TIMP-1 levels and the TIMP-1/MMP-1 ratio correlated negatively with peak VO2. They also described higher baseline peak VE/VCO2, TIMP-1, TIMP-1/MMP-1 ratio values, and lower MMP-1 levels in patients who suffered endpoints (total mortality, readmissions for heart failure, and cardiac transplantation). On multivariate analysis, VE/VCO2, MMP-1 levels, and age were the only variables independently related to prognosis of these patients [31]. Similarly, detectable plasma levels of MMP-13 were reduced in patients with LV hypertrophy and HF [32]. Interestingly, transgenic expression of human MMP-1 in mice (this MMP type is absent in rodents) and induction of LV pressure overload resulted in a relative reduction in myocardial fibrillar collagen content and improved indices of LV function [33]. These findings suggest that the loss of normal constitutive levels of certain MMP types, or failure of an induction of certain MMP types with LV pressure overload, may facilitate abnormal ECM accumulation and adverse myocardial remodeling.

Study of Morishita et al. demonstrated that in patients with heart failure with preserved ejection fraction (HFpEF), levels of BNP and the MMP-9/TIMP-1 ratio were lower compared to those with heart failure with reduced ejection fraction (HFrEF). An imbalance in the MMP/TIMP ratio and a robust increase in BNP levels reflect advanced ventricular remodeling, dilatation, and wall stretching. MMP and TIMP levels were similar in HFrEF and HFpEF patients and may represent ongoing myocardial injury and extracellular matrix remodeling before an increase in BNP and a decreased ejection fraction are seen. HFpEF is characterized by matrix apposition and myocardial stiffening [34]. Similarly, Martos et al. studied hypertensive patients divided into groups according to the presence of HFpEF and phase of diastolic function. Serum carboxy-terminal telopeptide of procollagen type I, carboxy-terminal telopeptide of procollagen type I, amino-terminal propeptide of procollagen type III, MMP-2, and MMP-9 levels were greater in patients with HFpEF than in those without. When controlled for age and gender, levels of serum carboxy-terminal telopeptide of procollagen type I, tissue inhibitor of MMP-1, amino-terminal propeptide of procollagen type III, concentrations of PICP (carboxy-terminal telopeptide of procollagen type I), and MMP-2 were increased in more severe phases of diastolic dysfunction. Within phases of diastolic dysfunction, markers of collagen production (such as serum carboxy-terminal telopeptide of procollagen type I, amino-terminal propeptide of procollagen type III) and MMP-2 and MMP-9 were elevated in those with HFpEF compared to those without signs of heart failure. Thus, a matrix and fibrosis markers such as MMPs may also be an important prognostic markers in HFpEF [35].

On the other hand, many clinical studies have quantified various circulating levels of MMPs and TIMPs in patients with HFrEF. MMP-8 levels were decreased in HF patients compared to controls [36]. The circulating levels of gelatinases, MMP-2, and MMP-9 have also been well characterized in HF patients. MMP-2 levels were elevated in HFrEF patients when compared to healthy controls and were correlated with LV volume, fractional shortening, and NYHA classifications [37–40]. Furthermore, MMP-2 levels were an independent predictor of mortality in patients with HFrEF [38]. Similarly, clinical studies have reported elevated circulating MMP-9 levels in SHF patients compared to healthy controls [41], but, by contrast, there are also reports that there are no differences between circulating levels of MMP-9 in SHF and control groups [37]. The discrepancies between these studies are not explained by variations in severity, HF etiology, or age. MMP-3 levels were increased in patients with SHF due to dilated cardiomyopathy and were correlated negatively with changes in the LV dimensions and volume, and independently predictive for cardiac events (death and hospitalization) [42]. In addition, MMP-3 levels were increased in patients after acute myocardial infarction who developed CHF [43].

3.3. MMPs in acute coronary syndromes

Acute coronary syndrome (ACS) is a term used for a group of conditions due to decreased blood flow in the coronary arteries such that part of the heart muscle is unable to act properly or dies. ACS is one of the leading causes of cardiovascular death. It includes unstable angina (UA), non-ST segment elevation myocardial infarction (NSTEMI), and myocardial infarction with ST segment elevation (STEMI) [44]. Most cases of ACS are caused by the erosion or rupture of an atherosclerotic plaque, a thickening of the vessel wall in a coronary artery with consequential thrombus formation. ACS is one of the leading causes of cardiovascular death, and early diagnosis of ACS is important because of the improvement in prognosis following timely interventions. It seems that some matrix metalloproteinases are implicated in the pathogenesis of cardiovascular diseases. Inflammatory components also appear to be correlated with development of atherosclerosis and ACS [45].

Hamed and Fattah measured levels of MMP-9 as a potential risk factor in 75 patients with ACS compared to 25 patients with stable angina (SA) and 20 healthy participants. In this study, patients in the SA group had significantly lower MMP-9 levels than those with ACS. Patients with ST-elevated myocardial infarction (MI) had highest MMP-9 levels, while in the control group, the lowest levels of MMP-9 were found. Patients with ACS having poor disease outcome (recurrent ischemic attacks, congestive heart failure, or death) had significantly higher MMP-9 levels. Cutoff value of MMP-9 equal to 3100 pg./mL was able to discriminate MI from unstable angina (UA). The best prognostic utility for MMP-9 was established at 4700 pg./mL [46].

Kai et al. reported that circulating MMP-2 and MMP-9 levels on admission were elevated in patients with acute myocardial infarction (AMI) and UA [47]. Inokubo et al. also reported that coronary circulation plasma concentrations of MMP-9 were significantly higher in the in-patients with AMI and UA when compared to control subjects. This finding supposes a process of active plaque rupture in acute coronary syndrome [48]. Hirohata et al. and Hojo et al. also observed increased concentrations of plasma MMP-1 and MMP-2 in patients with acute myocardial infarction [49, 50]. In the last ESC guidelines for the management of acute coronary syndromes in patients presenting without persistent ST-segment elevation, determination of concentrations of high-sensitive troponin T in the short "rule-in"/"rule-out" algorithms is recommended in the early diagnostic of ACS [51]. In the ACS, both MMP-9 and TnT levels are elevated compared to the control group. But, Kobayashi et al. have shown that within 4 h of ACS onset only the plasma level of MMP-9 was markedly increased. By contrast, concentrations of TnT were not significantly altered. In addition, MMP-9 concentrations were significantly higher in patients within first hours of ACS than in patients with late ACS independent of having STEMI or NSTEMI. On the contrary, levels of hs-TnT were significantly lower in patients with early ACS than with late ACS. This study indicates that plasma levels of MMP-9 increase approximately 80 minutes after the onset of ACS and sustain for 24 h thereafter. On the other hand, serum levels of hs-TnT peaked at 12–24 h after ACS onset [52].

The long-term study from Dhillon et al. examined the predictive value for cardiac events (death, readmission with HF, or recurrent MI) of MMP-2, MMP-3, and MMP-9 levels in patients with acute coronary syndrome in comparison to established markers, e.g. N-terminal pro-B-type natriuretic peptide (NT-proBNP) and the Global Registry of Acute Coronary Events (GRACE) score. In this study, MMP-2 and MMP-3 were elevated in patients with fatal outcome compared to survivors but were similar in patients with CHF or MI. MMP-9 levels were similar across study endpoints. Using Cox proportional hazards modeling, MMP-2 demonstrated an independent prediction of death with HR 6.60, along with NT-proBNP (HR 4.62) and the GRACE score (HR 1.03). MMP-3, MMP-9 levels, and log10-troponin I were not predictive for negative outcome. The areas under the receiver operating characteristic curves were 0.60 and 0.58 for MMP-2 and MMP-3, respectively, compared to 0.82 for NT-proBNP and 0.84 for the GRACE score (all statistically significant) for one-year mortality. Kaplan-Meier analysis showed that MMP-2 concentrations in the highest quartile were associated with higher mortality rates ($P = 0.006$, log rank 12.49). MMP-2 and MMP-3 levels revealed a weak association with HF readmission on univariate analysis, which was lost after adjustment for other clinical factors and situations. In this study, none of the MMPs tested predicted onset of MI [53].

As mentioned above, significant portion of regulation components for MMP production in the myocardium after the myocardial infarction is induced by the local proinflammatory cytokines. In an animal model of myocardial injury after AMI, the authors demonstrated that a local increase in TNF-α production in the myocardium is directly responsible for the increased production of local MMP-9 and MMP-2. This is associated with changes in transition of integrin isoforms, which can lead to such aggressive collagen dissolution that causes an acute myocardial rupture. If this process continues without rupture, heart walls become thick and significantly dilated, which leads to decreased function of the ventricle and poor survival. However, deletion of the gene for TNF-α through genetic manipulation in the host animal leads to a significant reduction in the concentrations of the inflammatory cytokines, which is associated with the reduction in local MMP activation. This results in a significant decrease in the incidence of heart wall rupture and a reduction in the subsequent heart size and development of heart failure with reduced ejection fraction of the LV [2]. Kelly et al. examined the temporal profiles of plasma concentrations of MMP-2 and MMP-9 and their relationship with echocardiographic parameters of left ventricle function and remodeling in humans after acute myocardial infarction. They showed that higher peak concentrations of plasma MMP-9 were associated with the extent of LV remodeling, which led to greater impairment of left ventricular function. In contrast, higher plateau levels of MMP-9 in the days after acute myocardial infarction were associated with a lesser degree of heart remodelation, and relative preservation of ventricular function [54].

3.3.1. Restenosis

The role of MMPs in iatrogenic postprocedural vasculopathy has also attracted a great deal of interest. The development of percutaneous coronary intervention (PCI) has provided a powerful means for treating ischemic heart disease. About 25–40% of patients undergoing PCI without a stent implantation have a recurrence of coronary artery disease symptoms within 6 months because of restenosis at the original site. A combination of events is involved in this pathological process, e.g. the migration and rapid growth of medial vascular smooth muscle cells, local production of chemocytokines, and other biologically active substances with formation of a characteristic lesion of fibrocellular intimal hyperplasia.

Hojo et al. investigated changes in MMP-2 levels in the coronary circulation after PCI in patients with angina pectoris. Plasma MMP-2 levels in the coronary sinus increased significantly 4 h after PCI. A positive correlation between concentrations of MMP-2 in the fourth hour after PCI and *late loss index* measured 6 months after PCI was observed. Authors suggested that excessively raised concentrations of MMPs in dilated coronary arteries after PCI lead to abnormal vascular remodeling and late restenosis by boosting migration of VSMCs and eventual formation of thrombus [55].

3.4. MMPs in atherosclerosis

It is widely accepted that atherosclerosis is promoted by mechanical and/or chemical injury of the vascular endothelium. This is followed by transendothelial migration of circulating monocytes from the circulating blood into the intima, where they become activated and produce a variety of cytokines, growth factors, and other biologically active substances. Formation of an atherosclerotic plaque occurs as a result of cellular migration and local proliferation followed by an accumulation of ECM, lipids, and calcium. Degradation of vascular ECM regulated by MMP-2 promotes smooth muscle cell migration and early plaque development. During the initial period of atherosclerotic plaque development, outward growth produces compensatory enlargement of the artery wall that involves matrix remodeling. Hypertension and aging lead to decrease of arterial compliance, which correlates with gradual accumulation of collagen and loss of elastin. In the latter stages of atherosclerotic process, disruption of the atherosclerotic plaque due to rupture of the fibrous cap or superficial erosion of the endothelium may occur followed by thrombotic complications. These processes (atherosclerotic plaque rupture and formation of thrombus) depend on excessive ECM degradation. Neovascularization of the atherosclerotic plaque may also play a role in destabilization of the plaque. The angiogenesis within the plaque is influenced and regulated by MMP activity through interactions between proteinases and integrins.

Extreme stage of arterial remodeling due to increased ECM degradation mediated by MMP-2 and MMP-9 is represented as aneurysm formation [56]. Some previous studies showed that lipid-laden macrophages infiltrating human atherosclerotic plaque produce MMP-1 and MMP-3. Culture of these macrophages with fibrous caps of human atherosclerotic plaque leads to MMP-dependent collagen cleaving [57]. Henney et al. found the presence of MMP-3 transcripts in atherosclerotic lesions from coronary arteries, which were localized together with clusters of lipid-laden macrophages in the shoulder areas of the atherosclerotic plaque [58]. Galis et al. reported that normal arteries and atherosclerotic plaque had different origins of MMPs. MMP-2 is secreted by VSMCs in all layers of nonatherosclerotic arteries, whereas in the atherosclerotic lesions, MMP-1, MMP-3, and MMP-9 production is localized to macrophages, VSMCs, and endothelial cells [59]. Some other studies have also reported the expression of several other MMPs including MMP-1, MMP-2, MMP-7, MMP-9, and MMP-12 in the shoulder areas of the plaque [60–62]. The demise of atherosclerotic plaque occurs through structural disruption of the arterial wall, which triggers thrombosis, the cause of occlusion and the majority of acute vascular events. The discovery of strong local MMP overexpression and in situ matrix-degrading activity in the vulnerable shoulders of human atheroma has provided a potential mechanistic insight into the process of plaque destabilization through matrix weakening by MMPs, especially in the vulnerable shoulders [63]. Resident macrophage-derived foam cells, characteristic of unstable plaques, have been identified as a major source of MMPs, including MMP-1, MMP-2, MMP-3, MMP-7, and MMP-associated activity in human and experimental atherosclerotic lesions [64].

It has been suggested that alternative ways or complementary systems for activation of latent MMPs in atherosclerotic plaques may exist. Purified Pro-MMP-2 can be activated in vitro by proteolytical activity of thrombin and this mechanism could provide cell-independent MMP activation at sites of vascular injury [65]. Another proteolytic-activating mechanism of MMP preforms may represent plasminogen cascade. Urokinase-type plasminogen activator (uPA) and plasminogen activator inhibitor-1 (PAI-1) can also contribute to the development of experimental neointimal lesions after injury and to aortic medial destruction, which was demonstrated in u-PA and PAI-1–null mice [66].

3.5. MMPs in cardiomyopathies

Cardiomyopathies (CMPs) are defined by structural and functional abnormalities of the ventricular myocardium that are unexplained by flow-limiting coronary artery disease or abnormal loading conditions. In the past, this group of diseases has been subdivided into primary CMP, in which the heart is the only involved organ, and secondary forms, where the cardiomyopathy represents a manifestation of other systemic disorders. Hypertrophic cardiomyopathy (HCM) is defined by the presence of increased left ventricular (LV) wall thickness that is not solely explained by abnormal loading conditions [67], or, in other words, hypertrophic cardiomyopathy (HCM) is defined morphologically as an unexplained hypertrophy in the absence of the reason for such a hypertrophy (e.g. hemodynamic stress). At the histological level is HCM characterized by myocyte disarray, fibrosis, and abnormalities of the intramyocardial small vessels. HCM represents a monogenic disease of the heart with an autosomal dominant way of heritability and different penetrance. Its prevalence in the general population is estimated in the rate of 1/500 [68]. Impaired collagenolysis and an increased deposition of collagen have been seen in patients with HCM. A significant reduction of MMP-1, practically to undetectable levels, was described in the patients with HCM. On the contrary, an increase of MMP-2 and MMP-9 concentration was found in these patients [69]. Described changes in MMP levels result in augmented ECM turnover, characterized by an increase of collagen type I and a shift of collagen I to collagen III production. This shift is not easy to explain because collagen I is patently more rigid than collagen III. This situation could be a compensatory mechanism due to the increase in wall stiffness [70]. Activity of MMP-2 in heart failure with preserved ejection fraction correlates negatively with systolic function of left ventricle and its levels are significantly rising with higher NYHA functional class. In the study of Noji et al., the plasma concentrations of MMP-2, MMP-3, MMP-9, TIMP-1, and TIMP-2 in patients with systolic dysfunction defined as fractional shortening (FS) <25% (group A), linked to HCM, in patients with HCM without systolic dysfunction (FS ≥ 25%; group B), and in healthy control subjects who were age-matched were measured. The concentration of MMP-2 in group A was significantly higher than in group B and the control subjects, whereas there was no significant difference between group B and the control subjects. MMP-2 concentrations significantly increased as the NYHA functional class increased in patients with HCM. MMP-3 and MMP-9 concentrations did not differ among the 3 groups. Both MMP-2 and TIMP-2 correlated significantly with FS and LV dimension, negatively and positively, respectively [71].

The best-known cardiac disease with respect to myocardial MMP activity is dilated cardiomyopathy (DCM). A characteristic feature of the DCM is an increase in left ventricle radius to wall thickness, which increases myocardial wall stress. This leads to further dilation and closes "circulus vitiosus." The etiology of DCM can be divided into ischemic (50–70%) and nonischemic (30–50%), with the latter phenotype including genetic and acquired causes [72]. In Western countries, 20–50% of DCM patients have evidence for familial disease. In animal and human studies in dilated cardiomyopathy, an increase in collagen type I and III production and deposition has been reported, so the collagen type I/type III ratio is constantly increased. As mentioned above, collagen type I is more "rigid" as collagen type III, providing more tensile strength and resulting in a stiffer matrix. As the left ventricle wall gets thicker during the progression of DCM, excessive production of collagen is considered to be an effort to strengthen the heart wall. More core matrix components are overproduced within the DCM-stricken myocardium, including elastin, laminin, and tenascin C. Furthermore, in the DCM heart arise a new complex interplay between various MMPs and TIMPs. This for example includes the MMPs present within the cardiovascular tissue (MMP-1, MMP-2, and MMP-9) and all four known TIMPs. Animal studies and models show that the enhanced MMP production and protein abundance occur with the initiation of LV dilation, and it might be a very early event in DCM. Progression of DCM is characterized by a decrease in MMP activity, due to an increase in TIMPs production [73]. In a study by Rouet-Benzineb et al., it was demonstrated that MMP-2 and MMP-9 activities were increased in DCM. In this study, MMP-2 levels were significantly increased not only within the myocardial interstitium, but also in cardiocytes. As showed before, MMP-2 may also cleave contractile proteins, e.g. myosin. Thus, increased MMP levels within the myocardium of patients with DCM may have multiple negative consequences that include matrix degradation and proteolytic activation of biologically active signaling molecules and degradation of contractile structures and, finally, directly affect myocyte structure and function [74].

4. Future directions

Ongoing studies targeting receptors for the ECM components have shown potential for new, targeted therapeutics, including several in various stages of clinical trials. Specific ECM proteins interact with cells and play an active role in intercellular signaling to control cell behavior that is critical to the repair or fibrotic process. Effective antifibrotic therapies would be a significant contribution in the treatment of some cardiac diseases as well as many other fibrotic diseases. Strategies reducing overexpression of MMPs in heart diseases may modify the development (or the speed of development) of adverse cardiac remodeling and, e.g., onset of the heart failure after myocardial infarction. This concept has indeed been proved in several basic studies, particularly with the inhibition of MMP-9, which represents one of the major MMPs involved in myocardial remodeling. Most of these studies show improvement in ventricular function and a reduction in ventricular size after administration of the MMP inhibitors [75]. Unfortunately, administration of various MMP inhibitors led to adverse events and number of leading candidates for the therapy have been withdrawn from development for this indication because of onset of fibromyalgia side effects in earlier trials attempting to decrease metastasis in cancer. Pharmacologic strategies affecting upstream signaling cascades involved in MMP transcription and regulation can participate in the process of our understanding of the complex myocardial remodeling and the specific role of MMPs and TIMPs. For example, the use of cytokine inhibition in biological therapy (such as administration of tumor necrosis factor-α neutralizing proteins) may prove to be useful pharmacological tools in order to identify the signaling pathways obligatory for MMP species induction [76].

On the other hand, many of the currently used treatment strategies may already partially affect MMP activation pathways as part of their "modus operandi." For example, part of the benefit of treatments such as acetylsalicylic acid or statins may decrease the cytokine and inflammatory response and so limit the bioactivity of MMPs.

Tissue engineering may open new avenues to create intelligent scaffolds to support regeneration of diseased or damaged tissue.

Author details

Marek Pytliak*, Viliam Vaník and Peter Bojčík

*Address all correspondence to: marek.pytliak@svetzdravia.com

Hospital of arm. gen. L. Svoboda a.s., Svidník, Slovakia

References

[1] Weber KT. Cardiac interstitium in health and disease: The fibrillar collagen network. Journal of the American College of Cardiology. 1989;**13**(6):1637-1652

[2] Liu P, Sun M, Sader S. Matrix metalloproteinases in cardiovascular disease. The Canadian Journal of Cardiology. 2006;**22**(Suppl B):25B-30B

[3] Horn MA, Trafford AW. Aging and the cardiac collagen matrix: Novel mediators of fibrotic remodelling. Journal of Molecular and Cellular Cardiology. 2016;**93**:175-185. DOI: 10.1016/j.yjmcc.2015.11.005

[4] Weber KT, Sun Y, Bhattacharya SK, Ahokas RA, Gerling IC. Myofibroblast mediated mechanisms of pathological remodelling of the heart. Nature Reviews. Cardiology. 2013;**10**:15-26

[5] Porter KE, Turner NA. Cardiac fibroblasts: At the heart of myocardial remodeling. Pharmacology & therapeutics. 2009;**123**(2):255-278 Epub May 23, 2009

[6] Lenkiewicz JE, Davies MJ, Rosen D. Collagen in human myocardium as a function of age. Cardiovascular Research. 1972;**6**:549-555

[7] Bou-Gharios G, Ponticos M, Rajkumar V, Abraham D. Extra-cellular matrix in vascular networks. Cell Proliferation. 2004;**37**(3):207-220. DOI: 10.1111/j.1365-2184.2004.00306.x.

[8] Medugorac I. Characterization of intramuscular collagen in mammalian left ventricle. Basic Research in Cardiology. 1982;**77**(6):589-598

[9] Valiente-Alandi I, Schafer AE, Blaxall BC. Extracellular matrix-mediated cellular communication in the heart. Journal of Molecular and Cellular Cardiology. 2016;**91**:228-237. DOI: 10.1016/j.yjmcc.2016.01.011

[10] Mooney A, Jackson K, Bacon R, Streuli C, Edwards G, Bassuk J, et al. Type IV collagen and laminin regulate glomerular mesangial cell susceptibility to apoptosis via beta(1) integrin- mediated survival signals. The American Journal of Pathology. 1999;**155**:599-606

[11] Sanders MA, Basson MD. Collagen IV regulates Caco-2 cell spreading and p130Cas phosphorylation by FAK-dependent and FAK-independent pathways. Biological Chemistry. 2008;**389**:47-55

[12] Dostal D, Glaser S, Baudino TA. Cardiac fibroblast physiology and pathology. Comprehensive Physiology. 2015;**5**:887-909

[13] Turner NA, Porter KE. Regulation of myocardial matrix metalloproteinase expression and activity by cardiac fibroblasts. IUBMB Life. 2012;**64**:143-150

[14] Gabbiani G, Ryan GB, Majne G. Presence of modified fibroblasts ingranulation tissue and their possible role in wound contraction. Experientia. 1971;**27**:549-550

[15] Davis J, Molkentin JD. Myofibroblasts: Trust your heart and let fate decide. Journal of Molecular and Cellular Cardiology. 2013;**70**:9-18. DOI: 10.1016/j.yjmcc.2013.10.019.

[16] Matrisian LM. Metalloproteinases and their inhibitors in matrix remodeling. Trends in Genetics. 1990;**6**:121-125

[17] Lockhart M, Wirrig E, Phelps A, Wessels A. Extracellular matrix and heart development. Birth defects research Part A, Clinical and molecular Teratology. 2011;**91**:535-550

[18] Overall CM. Matrix metalloproteinase substrate binding domains, modules and exosites. Matrix Metalloproteinase Protocols. 2001;**151**:79-120

[19] Hijova E. Matrix metalloproteinasis: Their biological functions and clinical implication. Bratislavské Lekárske Listy. 2005;**106**(3):127-132

[20] Klein T, Bischoff R. Physiology and pathophysiology of matrix metalloproteases. Amino Acids. 2011;**41**(2):271-290. DOI: 10.1007/s00726-010-0689-x

[21] Fan D, Takawale A, Lee J, Kassiri Z. Cardiac fibroblasts, fibrosis and extracellular matrix remodeling in heart disease. Fibrogenesis & Tissue Repair. 2012;**5**:15-20

[22] Biolo A, Fisch M, Balog J, Chao T, Schulze PC, Ooi H, Siwik D, Colucci WS. Episodes of acute heart failure syndrome are associated with increased levels of troponin and extracellular matrix markers. Circulation: Heart Failure. 2010;**3**(1):44-50. DOI: 10.1161/CIRCHEARTFAILURE.108.844324 Epub Oct 22, 2009

[23] Shirakabe A, Asai K, Hata N, Yokoyama S, Shinada T, Kobayashi N, Mizuno K. Clinical significance of matrix metalloproteinase (MMP)-2 in patients with acute heart failure. International Heart Journal. 2010;**51**(6):404-410

[24] Hadipurnomo S, Setianto BY, Dinarti LK. Correlation of serum levels of matrix metalloproteinase-9 to acute heart failure event as a complication AF acute coronary syndrome. Acta Cardiologia Indonesiana. 2015;**1**:8-12

[25] Jong GP, Ma T, Chou P, Chang MH, Wu CH, Lis PC, Lee SD, Liu JY, Kuo WW, Huang CY. Serum MMP-9 activity as a diagnosing marker for the developing heart failure of post MI patients. The Chinese Journal of Physiology. 2006;**49**(2):104-109

[26] Tziakas DN, Chalikias GK, Hatzinikolaou HI, Stakos DA, Papanas N, Tentes IK, Kortsaris AX, Maltezos E, Hatseras DI, Kaski JC. Levosimendan use reduces matrix metalloproteinase-2 in patients with decompensated heart failure. Cardiovascular Drugs and Therapy. 2005;**6**:399-402

[27] Spinale FG, Coker ML, Heung LJ, Bond BR, Gunasinghe HR, Etoh T, Goldberg AT, Zellner JL, Crumbley AJ. A matrix metalloproteinase induction/activation system exists in the human left ventricular myocardium and is upregulated in heart failure. Circulation. 2000;**102**(16):1944-1949

[28] López B, González A, Querejeta R, Larman M, Díez J. Alterations in the pattern of collagen deposition may contribute to the deterioration of systolic function in hypertensive patients with heart failure. Journal of the American College of Cardiology. 2006;**48**:89-96

[29] Thomas CV, Coker ML, Zellner JL, Handy JR, Crumbley AJ, Spinale FG. Increased matrix metalloproteinase activity and selective upregulation in LV myocardium from patients with end-stage dilated cardiomyopathy. Circulation. 1998;**97**:1708-1715

[30] George J, Patal S, Wexler D, Roth A, Sheps D, Keren G. Circulating matrix metalloproteinase-2 but not matrix metalloproteinase-3, matrix metalloproteinase-9, or tissue inhibitor of matrix metalloproteinase-1 predicts outcome in patients with congestive heart failure. American Heart Journal. 2005;**150**:484-487

[31] Jordan A, Roldan V, Garcia M, Monmeneu J, de Burgos FG, Lip GY, et al, Matrix metalloproteinase-1 and its inhibitor, TIMP-1, in systolic heart failure: Relation to functional data and prognosis. Journal of Internal Medicine 2007;**262:**385-392

[32] Ahmed SH, Clark LL, Pennington WR, Webb CS, Bonnema DD, Leonardi AH, McClure CD, Spinale FG, Zile MR. Matrix metalloproteinases/tissue inhibitors of metalloproteinases: Relationship between changes in proteolytic determinants of matrix composition and structural, functional, and clinical manifestations. Circulation. 2006;**113**(17):2089-96

[33] Foronjy RF, Sun J, Lemaitre V, D'Armiento JM. Transgenic expression of matrix metalloproteinase-1 inhibits myocardial fibrosis and prevents the transition to heart failure in a pressure overload mouse model. Hypertension Research. 2008;**31**:725-735

[34] Morishita T, Uzui R, Mitsuke Y, Amaya N, Kaseno K, Ishida K, Fukuoka Y, Ikeda H, Tama N, Yamazaki T, Lee JD, Tada H. Association between matrix metalloproteinase-9 and worsening heart failure events in patients with chronic heart failure. ESC Heart Failure. 2017. Published online in Wiley Online Library. Available from: wileyonlinelibrary.com. DOI: 10.1002/ehf2.12137

[35] Martos R, Baugh J, Ledwidge M, O'Loughlin C, Conlon C, Patle A, Donnelly SC, McDonald K. Diastolic heart failure: Evidence of increased myocardial collagen turnover linked to diastolic dysfunction. Circulation. 2007;**115**(7):888-895

[36] Wilson EM, Gunasinghe HR, Coker ML, et al. Plasma matrix metalloproteinase and inhibitor profiles in patients with heart failure. Journal of Cardiac Failure. 2002;**8**:390-398

[37] Noji Y, Shimizu M, Ino H, et al. Increased circulating matrix metalloproteinase-2 in patients with hypertrophic cardiomyopathy with systolic dysfunction. Circulation Journal. 2004;**68**:355-360

[38] Radauceanu A, Ducki C, Virion JM, et al. Extracellular matrix turnover and inflammatory markers independently predict functional status and outcome in chronic heart failure. Journal of Cardiac Failure. 2008;**14**:467-474

[39] George J, Patal S, Wexler D, Roth A, Sheps D, Keren G. Circulating matrix metalloproteinase-2 but not matrix metalloproteinase-3, matrix metalloproteinase-9, or tissue inhibitor of metalloproteinase-1 predicts outcome in patients with congestive heart failure. American Heart Journal. 2005;**150**:484-487

[40] Klappacher G, Franzen P, Haab D, et al. Measuring extracellular matrix turnover in the serum of patients with idiopathic or ischemic dilated cardiomyopathy and impact on diagnosis and prognosis. The American Journal of Cardiology. 1995;**75**(14):913-918

[41] Kelly D, Khan SQ, Thompson M, et al. Plasma tissue inhibitor of metalloproteinase-1 and matrix metalloproteinase-9: Novel indicators of left ventricular remodelling and prognosis after acute myocardial infarction. European Heart Journal. 2008;**29**(17):2116-24

[42] Ohtsuka T, Nishimura K, Kurata A, Ogimoto A, Okayama H, Higaki J. Serum matrix metalloproteinase-3 as a novel marker for risk stratification of patients with nonischemic dilated cardiomyopathy. Journal of Cardiac Failure. 2007;**13**:752-758

[43] Kelly D, Khan S, Cockerill G, et al. Circulating stromelysin-1 (MMP-3): A novel predictor of LV dysfunction, remodelling and all-cause mortality after acute myocardial infarction. European Journal of Heart Failure. 2008;**10**:133-139

[44] Studenčan M. Akútny koronárny syndróm. Košice: Media Group, s.r.o; 2006. p. 192

[45] Hackett D, Davies G, Chierchia S, Maseri A. Intermittent coronary occlusion in acute myocardial infarction. The New England Journal of Medicine. 1987;**317**:1055-1059

[46] Hamed GM, Fattah MF. Clinical relevance of matrix metalloproteinase 9 in patients with acute coronary syndrome. Clinical and Applied Thrombosis/Hemostasis. 2015;**21**(8): 705-711. DOI: 10.1177/1076029614567309

[47] Kai H, Ikeda H, Yasukawa H, Kai M, Seki Y, Kuwahara F, Ueno T, Sugi K, Imaizumi T. Peripheral blood levels of matrix metalloproteinases-2 and 9 are elevated in patients with acute myocardial syndrome. Journal of the American College of Cardiology. 1998;**32**:368-372

[48] Inokubo Y, Hanada H, Ishizaka H, Fukushi T, Kamada T, Okumura K. Plasma levels of matrix metalloproteinase-9 and tissue inhibitor of metalloproteinase-1 are increased in the coronary circulation in patients with acute coronary syndrome. American Heart Journal. 2001;**141**:211-217

[49] Hirohata S, Kusachi S, Murakami M, Murakami T, Sano I, Watanabe T, Komatsubara I, Kondo J, Tsuji T. Time dependent alterations of serum matrix metalloproteinase-1 and metalloproteinase-1 tissue inhibitor after successful reperfusion of acute coronary syndrome. Heart. 1997;**78**:278-284

[50] Hojo Y, Ikeda U, Ueno S, Arakawa H, Shimada K. Expression of matrix metalloproteinases in patients with acute myocardial infarction. Japanese Circulation Journal. 2001;**65**:71-75

[51] Task Force for the Management of Acute Coronary Syndromes in Patients Presenting without Persistent ST-Segment Elevation of the European Society of Cardiology (ESC). 2015 ESC Guidelines for the management of acute coronary syndromes in patients presenting without persistent ST-segment elevation. European Heart Journal. 2016;**37**:267-315

[52] Kobayashi N, Hata N, Kume N, Yokoyama S, Shinada T, Tomita K, et al. Matrix metalloproteinase-9 for the earliest stage acute coronary syndrome: Comparison with high-sensitivity troponin T. Circulation Journal. 2011;**75**:2853-2861

[53] OS1 D, Khan SQ, Narayan HK, Ng KH, Mohammed N, Quinn PA, Squire IB, Davies JE, Ng LL. Matrix metalloproteinase-2 predicts mortality in patients with acute coronary syndrome. Clinical Science (Lond). 2009;**118**(4):249-257. DOI: 10.1042/CS20090226

[54] Kelly D, Cockerill G, Thompson M, Khan S, Samani N, Squire I. Plasma metalloproteinase-9 and left ventriclar remodelling after acute myocardial infarction in man: a prospective cohort study. European Heart Journal. DOI: 10.1093/eurheartj/ehm003 Published online ahead of print Mar 5, 2007

[55] Hojo Y, Ikeda U, Katsuki T, Mizuno O, Fujikawa H, Shimada K. Matrix metalloproteinase expression in the coronary circulation induced by coronary angioplasty. Atherosclerosis. 2002;**161**:185-192

[56] Galis ZS, Khatri JJ. Matrix metalloproteinases in vascular remodeling and atherogenesis. The good, the bad, and the ugly. Circulation Research. 2002;**90**:251-262

[57] Shah PK, Falk E, Badimon JJ, Fernandez-Ortiz A, Mailhac A, Villareal-Levy G, Fallon JT, Regnstrom J, Fuster V. Human monocyte-derived macrophages induce collagen breakdown in fibrous caps of atherosclerotic plaques: Potential role of matrix-degrading metalloproteinases and implications for plaque rupture. Circulation. 1995;**92**: 1565-1569

[58] Henney AM, Wakeley PR, Davies MJ, Foster K, Hembry R, Murphy G, Humphries S. Localization of stromelysin gene expression in atherosclerotic plaques by in situ hybridization. Proceedings of the National Academy of Sciences of the United States of America. 1991;**88**:8154-8158

[59] Galis ZS, Sukhova GK, Lark MW, Libby P. Increased expression of matrix metalloproteinases and matrix degrading activity in vulnerable regions of human atheroslcerotic plaques. The Journal of Clinical Investigation. 1994;**94**:2493-2503

[60] Nikkari ST, O'Brien KD, Ferguson M, Hatsukami T, Welgus HG, Alpers CE, Clowes AW. Interstitial collagenase (MMP-1) expression in human carotid atherosclerosis. Circulation. 1995;**92**:1393-1398

[61] Halpert I, Sires UI, Roby JD, Potter-Perigo S, Wight TN, Shapiro SD, Welgus HG, Wickline SA, Parks WC. Matrilysin is expressed by lipid-laden macrophages at sites of potential rupture in atherosclerotic lesions and localizes to areas of versican deposition, a proteoglycan substrate for the enzyme. Proceedings of the National Academy of Sciences of the United States of America. 1996;**93**:9748-9753

[62] Shu YE, Humphries S, Henney A. Matrix metalloproteinases: Implication in vascular matrix remodeling during atherogenesis. Clinical Science. 1998;**94**:103-110

[63] Galis Z. Molecular mechanisms of plaque weakening and disruption. In: Brown D, editor. Cardiovascular Plaque Rupture. New York, NY: Marcel Dekker Inc.; 2002. p. 79-121

[64] Galis ZS, Sukhova GK, Kranzhöfer R, Clark S, Libby P. Macrophage foam cells from experimental atheroma constitutively produce matrixdegrading proteinases. Proceedings of the National Academy of Sciences of the United States of America. 1995;**92**:402-406

[65] Galis ZS, Kranzhofer R, Fenton JW, Libby P. Thrombin promotes activation of matrix metalloproteinase-2 produced by cultured vascular smooth muscle cells. Arteriosclerosis, Thrombosis, and Vascular Biology. 1997;**17**:483-489

[66] Carmeliet P, Moons L, Dewerchin M, Mackman N, Luther T, Breier G, Ploplis V, Muller M, Nagy A, Plow E, Gerard R, Edgington T, Risau W, Collen D. Insights in vessel development and vascular disorders using targeted inactivation and transfer of vascular endothelial growth factor, the tissue factor receptor, and the plasminogen system. Annals of the New York Academy of Sciences. 1997;**811**:191-206

[67] The Task Force for the Diagnosis and Management of Hypertrophic Cardiomyopathy of the European Society of Cardiology (ESC). 2014 ESC Guidelines on diagnosis and management of hypertrophic cardiomyopathy. European Heart Journal. 2014;**35**:2733-2779

[68] Cambronero F, Marı'n F, Rolda'n V, Hernandez-Romero D, Valde's M, Lip YM. Biomarkers of pathophysiology in hypertrophic cardiomyopathy: Implications for clinical management and prognosis. European Heart Journal. 2009;**30**:139-151

[69] Fassbach M, Schwartzkopff B. Elevated serum markers for collagen synthesis in patients with hypertrophic cardiomyopathy and diastolic dysfunction. Zeitschrift für Kardiologie. 2005;**94**:328-335

[70] Lombardi R, Betocchi S, Losi MA, Tocchetti CG, Aversa M, Miranda M, D'Alessandro G, Cacace A, Ciampi Q, Chiariello M. Myocardial collagen turnover in hypertrophic cardiomyopathy. Circulation. 2003;**108**:1455-1460

[71] Noji Y, Shimizu M, Ino H, Higashikata T, Yamaguchi M, Nohara A, Horita T, Shimizu K, Ito Y, Matsuda T, Namura M, Mabuchi H. Increased circulating matrix metalloproteinase-2 in patients with hypertrophic cardiomyopathy with systolic dysfunction. Circulation Journal. 2004;**68**:355-360

[72] Hershberger RE, Hedges DJ, Morales A. Dilated cardiomyopathy: the complexity of a diverse genetic architecture. Nature Reviews. Cardiology. 2013;**10**:531-547

[73] Louzao-Martinez L, Vink A, Harakalova M, Asselbergs FW, Verhaar MC, Cheng C. Characteristic adaptations of the extracellular matrix in dilated cardiomyopathy. International Journal of Cardiology. 2016;**220**:634-646

[74] Rouet-Benzineb P, Buhler JM, Dreyfus P, Delcourt A, Dorent R, Perennec J, Crozatier B, Harf A, Lafuma C. Altered balance between matrix gelatinases (MMP-2 and MMP-9) and their tissue inhibitors in human dilated cardiomyopathy: Potential role of MMP-9 in myosin-heavy chain degradation. European Journal of Heart Failure. 1999;**1**:337-352

[75] Rohde LE, Ducharme A, Arroyo LH, et al. Matrix metalloproteinase inhibition attenuates early left ventricular enlargement after experimental myocardial infarction in mice. Circulation. 1999;**99**:3063-3070

[76] Deswal A et al. Safety and efficacy of a soluble P75 tumor necrosis factor receptor (Enbrel, etanercept) in patients with advanced heart failure. Circulation. 1999;**99**:3224-3226

Chapter 3

Matrix Metalloproteinases MMP-3 and MMP-9 as Predictors of In-Stent Restenosis

Pavlina Kusnierova and Leos Pleva

Additional information is available at the end of the chapter

http://dx.doi.org/10.5772/intechopen.69589

Abstract

The present study aimed to demonstrate the use of matrix metalloproteinases (MMP-2, MMP-3 and MMP-9) as possible additional biochemical predictors of in-stent restenosis (ISR) and determined their reference intervals in adults with respect to gender and age. We included 111 consecutive patients treated at the cathlab of the University Hospital Ostrava, Czech Republic, with ISR within 12 months after implantation of a bare-metal stent. The control group consisted of 111 matched patients with identical main demographic and clinical risk factors. To set the reference intervals for MMPs, we measured the blood concentrations of these analytes in a group of healthy volunteers (N = 180) with an average age of 40–50 years. The enzyme concentrations were measured by immunosorbent assay. Statistical analysis was performed using IBM SPSS Statistics version 22 and MedCalc Version 14.12. We found that increased levels of MMP-3 and 9 were associated with a significant increase in ISR risk. The MMP-9 cut-off value for ISR risk prediction was determined to be ≥64.8 ng/mL. We suppose that screening of these biochemical parameters might be helpful to a more detailed risk stratification of patients after percutaneous coronary interventions, who would be able to benefit from implantation of drug-eluting stents.

Keywords: adult, age dependence, enzyme-linked immunosorbent assay, gender dependence, in-stent restenosis, matrix metalloproteinases

1. Introduction

Matrix metalloproteinases (MMPs) are members of a family of zinc-dependent proteolytic enzymes. The main function of MMPs is to degrade the various components of the extracellular matrix (ECM) and participate as regulators of extracellular tissue signalling networks. MMPs have broad substrate specificity and contribute to the homeostasis of many tissues and participate in several physiological processes, such as bone remodelling, angiogenesis, immunity and wound healing. MMPs are produced by activated inflammatory cells (neutrophils and macrophages) and wound cells (epithelial cells, fibroblasts and vascular endothelial cells). MMP activity is tightly regulated at the level of transcription, pro-peptide activation and inhibition by tissue inhibitors of MMPs (TIMPs).

The MMP process represents the procedure of pathologic changes in the tissues in atherosclerosis, arterial remodelling and myocardial repair following infarction [1]. A mechanical damage causes expression of matrix metalloproteinases (MMP), and it is proved that they may take part in the pathogenesis of in-stent restenosis (ISR), when undergoing coronary stent implantation by percutaneous coronary intervention [2–5].

Effectiveness of percutaneous coronary intervention (PCI) has remarkably become better after coronary stent implantation. Thanks to the early obstacles of plane balloon angioplasty that could be managed and in case the elastic recoil and constrictive remodelling has been applied, it comes to the reduction of the frequency of restenosis after PCI. Although these improvements have been implemented, a new complication has occurred in-stent restenosis (ISR) caused by neointimal hyperplasia. The clinical probability of occurrence of ISR after bare-metal stent implantation is about 20–35% [6, 7]. Additional decline of ISR occurrence to 5–10% has been caused by the usage of drug-eluting stents [6, 7]. Unfortunately, long-term dual antiplatelet therapy needs to be applied and is connected with the threat of late and very late stent thrombosis. The known predictors of ISR include patient-, vessel- and procedure-related agents [6, 7]. Because of not decreasing amount of patients going through PCI, there were strives to find other predisposing factors that would lead to more focused treatment.

2. Aims

We focused on matrix metalloproteinases (MMP-2, MMP-3 and MMP-9) as possible additional biochemical predictors of in-stent restenosis (ISR) after coronary artery bare-metal stenting and determined their reference intervals in adults with respect to gender and age.

3. Patient group and methods

Note that, 111 patients were recruited from the University Hospital Ostrava, Czech Republic affected by ISR within 12 months after implantation of a bare-metal stent. The control group (n = 111) with absent ISR 12 months after implantation of a bare-metal stent coincided with patients treated at our cathlab with identical main demographic and clinical risk factors (sex, age, diabetes mellitus and implanted stent diameter ±0.5 mm).

To set the reference intervals for MMP-2, MMP-3 and MMP-9, we measured the blood concentrations of these analytes in a group of 180 healthy adult volunteers attending the Blood

Centre of the University Hospital Ostrava. We measured MMP concentrations in heparin plasma. Plasma samples from each patient and healthy volunteers were stored at −80°C for 2–3 months after centrifugation at 2500 × *g* at 4°C for 6 min and in 2 aliquots of 2 mL. The measurement of enzyme concentrations was performed by immunosorbent assay (ELISA) (BioVendor-Laboratorni Medicina a.s., Brno, Czech Republic).

Selective coronarography was determined in a Siemens Axiom device (Forchheim, Germany) in a common way from the radial approach with 5 F diagnostic catheters and the contrast medium Iomeron 400. Quantitative coronary angiography was executed, and percent diameter stenosis (%DS) was figured out. ISR was observed as a diameter stenosis ≥50% in the stented segment.

Multi-slice CT coronarography was assessed in all patients in the Siemens Somatom Definition AS + device (Forchheim, Germany), a single-source CT scanner in a 128-slice configuration. The maximum intensity projection (MIP) reconstructions and automatic software vessel analysis were applied for assessment of the lumen. Homogeneous enhancement (from the visual point of view, similar to the CT attenuation in the reference vessels) inside the stent lumen was reported to be normal or without any relation to ISR [8].

Statistical analysis was performed using IBM SPSS Statistics version 22 (SPSS Inc., Chicago, IL, USA). Measured biochemical parameters were categorized according to reference values, which were calculated using MedCalc Version 14.12 (origin) [9, 10]. Parametric and non-parametric statistical methods were applied, as appropriate, using NCSS 2007 (origin) for calculations and R software for graphical displays. Potential outliers were evaluated by Cook's distance and partitioning of the data according to Harris and Boyd [11]. There were linkages between measurands, which were assessed using Spearman's rank correlation (r_s) or Pearson's product-moment correlation coefficients (r_p), respectively. What is more, correlation testing, the age dependence of MMP-2 and MMP-3 was examined using piecewise polynomial models (multiphase models) [12].

Continuous variables with non-normal distribution are presented as the median and range (minimum–maximum) and were compared using the non-parametric Mann-Whitney U test. Categorical variables were compared by the chi-square test. The difference between measured biochemical parameters of the study and control groups was analysed by the chi-square test. The assessment of potential consequences of other features on the association observed between the levels of individual markers and ISR was applied multiple logistic regression. A forward stepwise method was used to establish the most notable risk values for ISR. Diabetes mellitus and other possible confounding variables have been taken into consideration. The stating of the optimal cut-off values of biochemical criteria was applied the receiver operating characteristic (ROC) analysis in order to prognosticate in-stent restenosis.

The studied protocol complied with the declaration of Helsinki and was approved by the Ethics Committee of the University Hospital Ostrava, Czech Republic. Written informed consent was obtained from each participant.

4. Results

There have not been found any remarkable differences in the patients with ISR and the control group, as far as the main demographic factors (age, gender and body mass index) or clinical risk factors (diabetes mellitus) concerned. Same ranges of coronary disease (multi-vessel disease, acute coronary syndromes) and similar lesion characteristics (complex lesion B2/C and length and diameter (±0.5 mm) of implanted stents) have been proved in the groups. What is more, in both groups, mostly similar biochemical criteria have been found (creatinine, glucose, triglycerides, High-density lipoprotein (HDL) and hsCRP). Nevertheless, the ISR group showed particularly lower total cholesterol ($p = 0.016$) and Low-density lipoprotein (LDL) ($p = 0.001$), and notably higher NT-pro-BNP ($p = 0.010$), in comparison to the treatment group. **Table 1** shows the summary of plasma levels of matrix metalloproteinases in all groups [13].

To set the reference intervals for MMP-2, MMP-3 and MMP-9, we measured the blood concentration in a group of healthy volunteers with an average age of 40–50 years. Plasma MMP-2 levels in these population showed statistically significant age dependence ($r_p = 0.171$; $p = 0.02$; $r_s = 0.161$; $p = 0.034$). Therefore, we divided the tested file into two groups: ≤49 and >50 years. The medians of these age groups were significantly different from each other ($p = 0.001$; $z = 3.15$). MMP-3 plasma concentrations were found to be significantly correlated with age ($r_p = 0.355$; $p = 0.00007$; $r_s = 0{,}308$; $p = 0.0006$) as well as with gender ($p \leq 0.001$; $z > 3.0$). Because of this, there were created two groups of the probands, according to the age ≤47 and >47 years. The dependence of the measured values on gender showed to be crucial. Since, only a small amount of men in the group of ≤47 years took part in the survey, the reference range has not been taken into account for this group. No statistically significant changes could be observed in plasma MMP-9 levels in relation to age, but there was found a link with gender ($p = 0.014$; $z = 2.39$). Because of the fact that the z-value was lower than 3 and the data performed a non-Gaussian distribution, the distribution in separate age-dependence subgroups was figured out. The reference ranges are depictured in **Table 2**. **Table 3** presents an outline of the results [14].

Furthermore, we compared the levels of plasma of matrix metalloproteinases in ISR patients with the normal reference values of these markers in the healthy population.

The correlation between MMP-3, MMP-9 and the incidence of ISR with respect to diabetes mellitus was studied using a logistic regression analysis. It was shown that MMP-3 (OR: 1.013, 95% CI: 1.004–1.023, $p = 0.005$) and MMP-9 (OR: 1.014, 95% CI: 1.008–1.020, $p < 0.0001$) are significantly associated with the occurrence of ISR (**Table 4**).

Methods	In-stent restenosis	Controls
MMP-2 (ng/mL)	173.76 (122.18–248.40)	163.58 (113.57–247.85)
MMP-3 (ng/mL)	43.37 (26.66–72.74)	31.48 (23.14–53.16)
MMP-9 (ng/mL)	88.40 (53.80–131.7)	44.90 (25.56–79.90)

Note: Data are given as median (lower and higher quartiles).

Table 1. Plasma levels of measured parameters of all patients and matched controls [13].

Analyte	*N*	Age (year)	Gender	2.5th	90thconfidence interval	97.5th	90th confidence interval
MMP-2 (ng/mL)	180	35–62	Both	110.0	97.1–124.1	590.9	520.8–670.0
	111	35–49	Both	98.3	83.0–115.2	466.9	417.9–519.1
	62	50-62	Both	160.8	144.8–179.0	550.2	456.9–666.7
MMP-3 (ng/mL)	120	34–61	Both	12.49	11.20–13.86	39.37	36.19–42.72
	38	34–47	Female	11.11	9.24–13.15	29.91	26.49–33.53
	14[a]		Male	–	–	–	–
	22	48–61	Female	12.76	11.11–14.69	31.14	25.41–38.40
	46		Male	18.03	15.84–20.38	42.04	38.00–46.33
MMP-9 (ng/mL)	116	16–61	Both	27.63	24.55–30.99	103.06	92.85–114.06
	58	20–61	Female	24.83	20.93–29.25	98.82	84.28–115.27
	58	19–55	Male	33.37	29.47–37.77	108.67	93.01–126.8

[a] Reference interval cannot be calculated due to the small number of data.

Table 2. The gender- and age-dependent reference intervals of MMP-2, MMP-3 and MMP-9 (μg/l)—2.5th, 97.5th centile values and their 90th confidence intervals according to parametric statistical methods [14].

Analyte	Age dependence	Gender dependence
MMP-2	Yes	No
MMP-3	Yes	Yes
MMP-9	No	Yes

Table 3. Summary of results as regards age- and gender-dependence of MMP-2, MMP-3 and MMP-9 [14].

Analyte	OR	95% CI for OR	*p*
MMP-2	1.001	0.999–1.004	0.326
MMP-3	1.013	1.004–1.023	0.005
MMP-9	1.014	1.008–1.020	<0.0001

Note: OR is associated with a single-unit increase in the value of the parameter.

Table 4. Logistic regression analysis (separately for each parameter with adjustment for diabetes mellitus (DM)) [13].

The result of this study is also the finding that the decreased concentration of MMP-9 below the lower limit of the reference interval is associated with a significant reduction in the incidence of ISR (OR: 0.265, 95% CI: 0.121–0.582, $p = 0.001$). On the other hand, the increased concentration of MMP-9 above the upper limit of the reference interval is associated with an increase in the incidence of ISR (OR: 2.685; 95% CI: 1.344–5.366; $p = 0.005$). At the same time, the increased concentration of MMP-3 above the upper limit of the reference interval is linked with an increased incidence of ISR (OR: 2.502; 95% CI: 1.441–4.344; p = 0.001). In this case, a multivariate logistic regression analysis was also used. A step-by-step method was used to select the most important categorized parameters that are predictive of ISR, with DM modifications and individual categorized parameters. It was found that MMP-9 is the most important parameter in terms of ISR prediction (OR: 0.322; 95% CI: 0.122–0.854; p = 0.023), its decrease below the lower limit of the reference interval is connected with a decrease in ISR.

Based on receiver operating characteristic (ROC) analysis, the plasma abundance of MMP-9 may be considered the most suitable parameter for use in ISR risk prediction (**Table 5** and **Figure 1**). The following cut-off values for prediction of ISR were determined: MMP-9 ≥ 64.8 ng/mL with sensitivity 65.8 and specificity 65.8% (**Table 6**).

Analyte	AUC
MMP-2	0.525
MMP-3	0.605
MMP-9	0.715

Note: Parameters with AUC > 0.7 or > 0.75 are suitable for the in-stent restenosis prediction.

Table 5. ROC analysis; area under the curve (AUC) of all parameters [13].

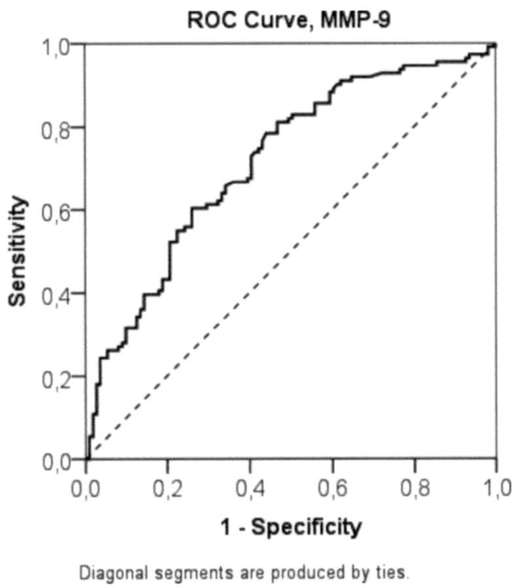

Figure 1. ROC curve of MMP-9 with AUC >0.7 is suitable for the ISR prediction [13].

Analyte	MMP-9	
AUC	0.715	
Cut-off value	≥64.8 (ng/mL)	
Sensitivity	65.8%	56.2–74.5%
Specificity	65.8%	56.2–74.5%
PPV	65.8%	56.2–74.5%
NPV	65.8%	56.2–74.5%
False positivities	34.2%	25.5–43.8%
False negativities	34.2%	25.5–43.8%

Table 6. Cut-off values of MMP-9 for ISR prediction [13].

5. Discussion

MMPs are a growing family of endopeptidases, they currently have at least 24 members, although some of them have not been well understood. Most of the MMPs contain a pro-peptide, a catalytic domain, a linker peptide and a hemopexin domain. MMPs are synthesized and secreted as latent pro-enzymes, containing a Zn^{2+}-binding active site and require Ca^{2+} for activation. MMPs are categorized by their structure and substrates into collagenases, gelatinases, stromelysins, matrilysins, membrane-type (MT)-MMPs and others. MMP-2 (gelatinase A) and MMP-9 (gelatinase B) are classified as a gelatinases, which degrade both collagens and gelatins [1].

MMP-2 and MMP-9 play an essential role in angiogenesis and arteriogenesis, two processes are critical to restoration of tissue perfusion after ischemia. MMP-2 expression is increased in tissue ischemia, but the responsible mechanisms remain unknown.

Expression and activity of MMPs are regulated at different levels: gene expression, proenzyme activation and enzyme secretion are inhibited specifically by tissue inhibitors of MMPs (TIMPs) and non-specifically alpha-2 macroglobulin. There is an increased expression of the genes encoding these proteins. Mutations of these genes are likely to affect the degree of expression, mRNA stability and the properties of the particular proteins, which may influence the process etiopathogenesis.

MMP-2 and MMP-9 are the most widely studied MMPs in blood vessel. MMP-3 (stromelysin-1) is included among stromelysins and is digested a wide range of extracellular matrix molecules and participated in proMMPs proteolysis. MMP-3 overexpression significantly reduces smooth muscle cells migration and inhibits neointimal formation in arterialized vein grafts. Ogata et al. reported that MMP-3 regulates vascular smooth muscle cells migration via MMP-9 activation. MMP-3 is already known as an activator of pro-MMP-9. Combination of MMP-3 and MMP-9 is required and efficient in neointimal hyperplasia [15–17].

Based on several published studies describing the discrepancies in MMP concentrations between serum and plasma [18–31], we measured MMP concentrations in heparin plasma. To set the reference intervals for MMP-2, MMP-3 and MMP-9, we measured the blood concentrations of these analytes in a group of healthy volunteers with an average age of 40–50 years. We found that plasma MMP-2 concentrations depend on the proband age (healthy volunteers). Lower MMP-2 concentrations were found in subjects <50 years of age and the concentration increased with age. However, no similar data were reported for a group of healthy volunteers.

The concentration of MMP-3 was statistically significant correlated with age and sex as well. The lower plasma concentrations of MMP-3 have been demonstrated in probes <47 years. MMP-3 concentrations in women were lower in both age groups than that in men.

Normal levels for MMP-3 determined by a one-step sandwich ELISA method with reagents provided by Dr Jaspar, Biosource Europe S. A., Belgium were described in 96 healthy controls (46 females and 50 males) in the study of Ribbens et al. [32, 33]. Our results showed higher plasma MMP-3 concentration in both women and men, as compared to Ribbens et al.'s data. The cause of this difference seems to be the use of different reagents.

Plasma MMP-9 concentrations are associated with difference in respect to gender. Our findings indicate lower values in women and higher in men. The publication of Lizasa et al. [34] also evaluated a group of healthy volunteers ($n = 138$). They used the plasma samples without any further specification of primary material and one-step sandwich enzyme immunoassay kit (Fuji Chemical Industries, Toyama, Japan) for their determination. Their results showed a common range of plasma MMP-9 concentration lower than our data and independent of gender or age. They also failed to mention the age variance of their healthy volunteers. It is found from other published studies that the measured concentrations of not only MMP-9 but also of other MMPs in blood are strongly influenced by the sampling procedure and by the type of used anticoagulant agent [18–31]. These reasons may stand for the found differences. Such differences in methodology could underlie the observed discrepancy between these studies.

These normal values were used for comparison of patients with in-stent restenosis after PCI and matched controls.

Percutaneous coronary intervention (PCI) is a rapid transduction of the coronary artery in most cases by means of a balloon catheter. Concomitant implantation of the coronary stent, which prevents the re-narrowing of the coronary artery, has reached a significant improvement in PCI. However, a new complication occurs: stent restenosis (ISR), developing from neointimal hyperplasia, which the basic element, is the transformation of smooth muscle cells from the contractile to the proliferative phenotype. The process of restenosis is initiated by endothelial denudation and deep vascular damage that starts adhesion and platelet activation. Activated platelets exclude growth factors that release smooth muscle cells from growth inhibition and induce their proliferation and subsequent migration from the media into the intimate. Proliferation of smooth muscle cells continues after the platelet phase. Activated smooth muscle cells themselves exclude growth factors that can affect the surrounding cells and help to maintain proliferation and migration. The second fundamental element of restenosis is the production and secretion of extracellular matrix by smooth muscle cells that migrated to the injured intimal zone. A complete neointimal layer can be observed already 2 weeks after implantation of the stent. Maximum restenosis is observed after 3–6 months and remains relatively stable after 1 year [6, 7].

To exclude ISR was used Multi-slice coronarography (MS-CT) coronarography due to non-invasiveness in the control group. Note that, 64- and more-slice MS-CT have almost 99% sensitivities and specificities for the detection of coronary artery stenoses in the native coronary arteries.

Visualization of the lumen inside the metal stents of the coronary artery by MS-CT is more demanding than the assessment of the native coronary artery with respect to the material used for stent manufacturing [35].

Sun [36] and Kumbhani [37] in their study described the advantages of MS-CT in detecting stent coronary restenosis (nearly 1400 and 1500 evaluated stents).

The sensitivity and specificity of MS-CT in detection of ISR were 90 and 91%, with positive and negative predictive values of 68 and 98%, respectively [36, 37].

In this study, the results of ISR patients were compared with those of the control group. Increased plasma concentrations of MMP-3 and MMP-9 were found to be significantly associated with a significant increase in ISR risk. The MMP-9 cut-off value for ISR risk prediction was determined to be ≥64.8 ng/ml. At the same time, no correlation between the MMP-2 values and the ISR occurrence has been demonstrated.

6. Conclusions

Age- and gender-specific reference intervals for heparin-plasma MMP-2, MMP-3 and MMP-9 were established based on a cohort of healthy subjects. Transference studies suggest that these intervals established by enzyme-linked immunosorbent assay are not comparable to published data mainly because of different type of used anticoagulant agent. In addition to this, each laboratory should have these reference intervals checked for its own population according to the Clinical and Laboratory Standards Institute (CLSI) guidelines.

At the same time, a statistically significant correlation has been demonstrated between increased MMP-3 and MMP-9 concentrations and an increased risk of ISR. For predicting the risk of ISR, the concentration of ≥ 64.8 ng/ml MMP-9 was determined. No correlation was demonstrated between MMP-2 concentration and ISR occurrence.

We suppose that screening of these biochemical parameters might be helpful to a more detailed risk stratification of patients after percutaneous coronary interventions, who would be able to benefit from implantation of drug-eluting stents.

Acknowledgements

This study was supported by Ministry of Health, Czech Republic—conceptual development of research organization—FNOs/2013 and by the project of European Social Fund and the State Budget of the Czech Republic, registration number CZ.1.07/2.3.00/20.0040.

Conflict of interest

The authors state that there are no conflicts of interest regarding the publication of this chapter.

Author details

Pavlina Kusnierova[1,2]* and Leos Pleva[3,4]

*Address all correspondence to: pavlina.kusnierova@fno.cz

1 Department of Biomedical Sciences, Faculty of Medicine, University of Ostrava, Ostrava, Czech Republic

2 Department of Clinical Biochemistry, Institute of Laboratory Medicine, University Hospital Ostrava, Ostrava, Czech Republic

3 Department of Cardiovascular Diseases, University Hospital Ostrava, Ostrava, Czech Republic

4 Department of Clinical Studies, Faculty of Medicine, University of Ostrava, Ostrava, Czech Republic

References

[1] Chen Q, Jin M, Yang F, Zhu J, Xiao Q, Zhang L. Matrix metalloproteinases: Inflammatory regulators of cell behaviors in vascular formation and remodeling. Mediators of Inflammation. 2013;**2013**:928315, 1-14. DOI: http://dx.doi.org/10.1155/2013/928315

[2] Ge J, Shen C, Liang C, Chen L, Qian J, Chen H. Elevated matrix metalloproteinase expression after stent implantation in associated with restenosis. International Journal of Cardiology. 2006;**112**(1):85-90

[3] Jones GT, Tarr GP, Philips LV, Wilkins GT, van Rija AM, Wiliams MJA. Active matrix metalloproteinases 3 and 9 are independently associated with coronary artery in-stent restenosis. Atherosclerosis. 2009;**207**(2):603-607

[4] Katsaros KM, Kastl SP, Zorn G, Maurer G, Wojta J, Huber K, Christ G, Speidl WS. Increased restenosis rate after implantation of drug-eluting stents in patients with elevated serum activity of matrix metalloproteinase 2 and 9. JACC: Cardiovascular Interventions. 2010;**3**(1):90-97

[5] Tarr GP, Williams GT, Wilkins VHT, Chenb LV, Phillips AM, van Rij AM, Jones GT. Intra-individual changes of active matrix metalloproteinase-9 are associated with clinical in-stent restenosis of bare metal stents. Cardiology. 2013;**124**:28-35

[6] Kim MS, Dean LS. In-stent restenosis. Cardiovascular Therapeutics. 2011;**29**(3):190-198

[7] Byrne RA, Joner M, Massberg S, Kastrati A. Restenosis in bare metal and drug-eluting stents. In: Escaned J, Serruys PW, editors. Coronary Stenosis, Imaging, Structure Anfphysiolohy. 1st ed. Toulouse, France: Europa Edition; 2010. pp. 475-496

[8] Sun Z, Davidson R, Lin CH. Multi-detector row CT angiography in the assessment of coronary in-stent restenosis: A systematic review. European Journal of Radiology. 2009;**69**(3):489-495

[9] Solberg HE. International Federation of Clinical Chemistry (IFCC). Scientific Committee, Clinical Section. Expert Panel on Theory of Reference Values (EPTRV) and International Committee for Standardization in Haematology (ICSH), Standing Committee on Reference Values. Approved recommendation (1987) on the theory of reference values. Part 5. Statistical treatment of collected reference values. Determination of reference limits. Journal of Clinical Chemistry and Clinical Biochemistry. 1987;**25**:645-656

[10] Horowitz GL, Altaie S, Boyd JC, Ceriotti F, Garg U, Horn P, Pesce A, Sine HE, Zakowski J. Clinical and Laboratory Standards Institute (CLSI). Defining, Establishing, and Verifying Reference Intervals in the Clinical Laboratory; Approved Guideline. CLSI D

[11] Harris EK, Boyd JC. On dividing reference data into subgroups to produce separate reference ranges. Clinical Chemistry. 1990;**36**(2):265-270

[12] Seber GAF, Wild CJ. Nonlinear regression. New York: John Wiley & Sons; 1989. DOI: ISBN 0471617601

[13] Pleva L, Kusnierova P, Plevova P, Zapletalova J, Karpisek M, Faldynova L, Kovarova P, Kukla P. Increased levels of MMP-3, MMP-9 and MPO represent predictors of in-stent restenosis, while increased levels of ADMA, LCAT, ApoE and ApoD predict bare metal stent patency Biomedical Paper Palacký University, Faculty of Medicine and Dentistry, Olomouc, Czech Republic. 2015;**159**(4):586-594. DOI: 10.5507/bp.2015.037. Epub 2015 Sep 3

[14] Kusnierova P, Vsiansky F, Pleva L, Plevova P, Safarcik K, Svagera Z. Reference intervals of plasma matrix metalloproteinases 2, 3, and 9 and serum asymmetric dimethylarginine levels. Scandinavian Journal of Clinical and Laboratory Investigation. 2015;**75**(6):508-513

[15] Kallenbach K, Salcher R, Heim A, Karck M, Mignatti P, Haverich A. Inhibition of smooth muscle cell migration and neointima formation in vein grafts by overexpression of matrix metalloproteinase-3. Journal of Vascular Surgery. 2009;**49**(3):750-758

[16] Ogata Y, Enghild JJ, Nagase H. Matrix metalloproteinase 3 (stromelysin) activates the precursor for the human matrix metalloproteinase 9. The Journal of Biological Chemistry. 1992;**267**(6):3581-3584

[17] Johnson JL, Dwivedi A, Somerville M, et al. Matrix metalloproteinase (MMP)-3 activates MMP-9 mediated vascular smooth muscle cell migration and neointima formation in mice. Arteriosclerosis, Thrombosis, and Vascular Biology. 2011;**31**(9):35-44

[18] Mannello F. Effects of blood collection methods on gelatin zymography of matrix metalloproteinases. Clinical Chemistry. 2003;**49**:339-340

[19] Kodama S, Iwata K, Iwata H, Yamashita K, Hayakawa T. Rapid one-step sandwich enzyme immunoassay for tissue inhibitor of metalloproteinases: An application for rheumatoid arthritis in serum and plasma. Journal of Immunological Methods. 1990;**127**:103-108

[20] Jung K, Nowak L, Lein M, Henke W, Schnorr D, Loening SA. Role of specimen collection in preanalytical variation of metalloproteinases and their inhibitors in blood. Clinical Chemistry. 1996;**46**:2043-2045

[21] Lein M, Nowak L, Jung K, Koenig F, Liuchtinghagen R, Schnorr D, Loening SA. Analytical aspects regarding the measurement of metalloproteinases and their inhibitors in blood. Clinical Biochemistry. 1997;**30**:491-496

[22] Jung K, Laube C, Lein M, Lichtinghagen R, Tschesche H, Schnorr D, Loening SA. Kind of sample as preanalytical determinant of matrix metalloproteinases 2 and 9 and tissue inhibitor of metalloproteinase 2 in blood. Clinical Chemistry. 1998;**44**:1060-1062

[23] Jung K, Lein M, Laube C, Lichtinghagen R. Blood specimen collection methods influence the concentration and the diagnostic validity of matrix metalloproteinase 9 in blood. Clinica Chimica Acta. 2001;**314**:241-244

[24] Jung K, Lein M, Roemer A, Lichtinghagen R. Circulating gelatinase B (MMP-9): The impact of preanalytical step of blood collection. Matrix Biology. 2002;**21**:381-382

[25] Alby C, Abdesselam OB, Foglietti MJ, Beaudeux JL. Preanalytical aspects regarding the measurement of metalloproteinase-9 and tissue inhibitor or metalloproteinase-1 in blood. Clinica Chimica Acta. 2002;**325**:183-186

[26] Mannello F, Luchetti F, Canonico B, Papa S. Effect of anticoagulants and cell separation media as preanalytical determinants on zymographic analysis of plasma matrix metalloproteinases. Clinical Chemistry. 2003;**49**:1956-1957

[27] John M, Jung K. Pre-analytical conditions for the assessment of circulating MMP-9 and TIMP-1: Consideration of pitfalls. The European Respiratory Journal. 2005;**26**:364-366

[28] Jung K, Meisser A, Bischof P. Blood sampling as critical preanalytical determinant to use circulating MMP and TIMP as surrogate markers for pathological processes. International Journal of Cancer. 2005;**116**:1000-1001

[29] Jung K, Gerlach RF, Tanus-Santos JE. Preanalytical pitfalls of blood sampling to measure true circulating matrix metalloproteinase 9 and tissue inhibitors of matrix metalloproteinases. Clinica Chimica Acta. 2006;**373**:180-181

[30] Jung K. Sample processing and its preanalytical impact on the measurement of circulating matrix metalloproteinases. Clinical Chemistry and Laboratory Medicine. 2006; **44**:500-502

[31] Jung K. Impact of blood sampling on circulating tissue inhibitors of metalloproteinases. Clinical Cancer Research. 2006;**12**:2648

[32] Ribbens C, Martiny Porras M, Franchimont N, Kaiser MJ, Jaspar JM, Damas P, Houssiau FA, Malaise MG. Increased matrix metalloproteinase-3 serum levels in rheumatic diseases: Relationship with synovitis and steroid treatment. Annals of the Rheumatic Diseases. 2002;**61**:161-166

[33] Brennan FM, Browne KA, Green PA, Jaspar JM, Maini RN, Feldmann M. Reduction of serum matrix metalloproteinase 3 in rheumatoid arthritis patients following anti-tumor necrosis factor-a (cA2) therapy. British Journal of Rheumatology. 1997;**36**:643-650

[34] Lizasa T, Fujisawa T, Suzuki M, Motohashi S, Yasufuku K, Yasukawa T, Baba M, Shiba M. Elevated levels of circulating plasma matrix metalloproteinase 9 in non-small cell lung cancer patients. Clinical Cancer Research. 1999;**5**:149-153

[35] Rixe J, Achenbach S, Ropers D, Baum U, Kuettner A, Ropers U, Bautz W, Daniel WG, Anders K. Assessment of coronary artery stent restenosis by 64-slice multi-detector computed tomography. European Heart Journal. 2006;**27**:2567-2572

[36] Sun Z, Marzouq A, Almutairi D. Diagnostic accuracy of 64 multislice CT angiography in the assessment of coronary in-stent restenosis: A meta-analysis. European Journal of Radiology. 2010;**73**:266-273

[37] Kumbhani DJ, Ingelmo CP, Schoenhagen P, Curtin RJ, Flamm SD, Desai MY. Meta-analysis of diagnostic efficacy of 64-slice computed tomography in the evaluation of coronary in-stent restenosis. American Journal of Cardiology. 2009;**103**:1675-1681

Section 3

Eye Disorders and Matrix Metalloproteinases

Chapter 4

Influence of Matrix Metalloproteinases MMP-2, -3 and on Age-Related Macular Degeneration Development

Rasa Liutkeviciene, Vykintas Liutkevicius,
Agne Giedraitiene, Loresa Kriauciuniene and
Virginija Asmoniene

Additional information is available at the end of the chapter

http://dx.doi.org/10.5772/intechopen.70551

Abstract

Age-related macular degeneration (AMD) is the leading cause of significant and irreversible central visual loss as it affects a small area of the retina, called the macula. However, the pathogenesis of still fairly understood. AMD has a multifactorial etiology, and its development might be influenced by body peculiarities, environmental and genetic factors. Risk factors such as age, gender, cigarette smoking, color of iris, nutrition, body mass index, oxidative stress, and genetic factors (complement factor H gene, Apo E gene, matrix metalloproteinases (MMPs) genes and others) increase probability to develop AMD. Here, we discuss about choroidal neovascularization process, where hypoxia, inflammatory process, and proteolytic enzymes play a main role, but mainly we focus on the family of matrix metalloproteinases (MMPs), especially on MMP -2, -3 and -9, and their impact on AMD development. MMPs belong to a family of proteolytic zinc-containing enzymes, and their mechanism under normal physiological conditions is precisely regulated, but when is dysregulated, MMPs become a cause of various diseases, including and AMD. MMPs are capable of degrading most of the extracellular matrix components, which are important in the remodeling during angiogenesis. Angiogenesis is the main pathological process associated with age-related macular degeneration development. Activated endothelial cells release MMPs which by degrading the basilar membrane allows capillaries to grow beneath the retina and retinal layers. Such capillaries often bleed, more liquids are filtered through the walls, and fibrous tissue grows within. Furthermore, swelling of the retina and impaired vision occur. In this book chapter, we focus on AMD prevalence, risk factors, clinics, diagnostics and influence of MMP-2, -3 and -9 on AMD development.

Keywords: AMD prevalence, risk factors, influence of MMP-2, -3 and -9

1. Introduction

Age-related macular degeneration (AMD) is a multifactorial disorder influenced by interaction between genetic and environmental risk factors. The most important pathogenetic mechanisms which cause AMD are the formation of drusen, hypoxia, local inflammation, and later, neovascularization. The development of neovascularization, mainly induced by retinal hypoxia, is a hallmark of AMD and its blockade has been considered as an inhibition of AMD development. Tissue ischemia leads to an increased secretion of the vascular endothelial growth factor (VEGF) and higher expression of the VEGF receptor 2. Vasodilatation induced by VEGF enhances vascular permeability and protease activity that results in developing and expansion of vascular network of the surrounding tissues and its remodeling [1, 2]. The fragmentation of a basilar membrane and an intracellular connective tissue are essential for the formation of new capillaries. Activated endothelial cells release various enzymes such as matrix metalloproteinases (MMPs) which degrade the basilar membrane, allowing capillaries to grow beneath the retina and between retinal layers. MMPs, which are found in all organisms, are endopeptidases which contain an active site Zn^{2+} and are divided into subfamilies of clans based on evolutionary relationships and structure of the catalytic domain. MMPs comprise a family of currently 25 related, yet distinct vertebrate gene products, of which 24 are found in mammals [3, 4]. MMPs are mainly classified into collagenases (MMP-1, -8, -13), gelatinases (MMP-2, -9), stromelysins (MMP-3, -10), membrane-type MMPs (MMP-14, -15, -16, -17), and others [2, 4].

2. Prevalence of age-related macular degeneration

All researchers agree that AMD is the most common cause of blindness in developed countries [1, 2]. The Lithuanian Medical Social Expertise Commission announced that in 2002, there were 13.8% of blind people due to AMD in Lithuania. The Blind Register Center reported that in Great Britain, nearly 50% of people live with blindness caused by AMD [5]. More than 30% of adults aged 75 years or older have AMD, and in about 6–8% of them, the disease would progress and cause the most severe visual loss [2]. Epidemiological studies in Australia, Europe and North America showed that the prevalence of AMD in the group of 55- to 64-year-old patients is about 0.2% and it increases to 13% in 85 years old patients group [3]. Studies showed that AMD can be diagnosed for people even younger than 40 years old [6]. The prevalence of AMD in a black population was 2.4%, in Spanish—4.2%, in Chinese—4.6%, and in whites—5.4% ($p < 0,001$, statistically significant between all groups). The highest prevalence of AMD is determined in 75–84 years old patients group, and it may vary from 7.4% (in a black population) to 15.8% (in white and Chinese populations) ($p = 0.03$). Additionally, it was reported that prevalence of the late AMD in a black population was 0.3%, in a Spanish population—0.2%, in Whites—0.6% and in Chinese population—1.0%. Several studies revealed that AMD was diagnosed in 8.5% of 43–54 year old population, while in patients over 75 years old—37% of AMD cases were diagnosed [7]. It is predicted that from 1980 to 2020, the elderly population in the developed countries and the developing countries will increase by

186 and 356%, respectively [1]. It was stated that older age is a natural risk factor for development of AMD; thus, blindness might experience increasing numbers in the older population. The World Health Organization predicts that in 2020, in the population over 60 years of age, the number of people with vision loss due to eye and vision-related problems would reach approximately 54 million [1]. Older blind or visually impaired persons are increasing in numbers as the population over the world is growing very rapidly. Today, there are over 6 billion people and by 2020, the population all over the world might reach up to 8 billion. Additionally, this increases a life expectancy of women and men, especially in the developing countries. It is predicted that during next 20 years, the population of people over 60 years of age will double from 400 to 800 million in the world [5].

3. Risk factors for age-related macular degeneration development

Various risk factors (modifiable and non-modifiable) such as smoking, obesity, age, gender, and others are associated with AMD development. Epidemiological studies have shown that genetic predisposition, systemic factors, lifestyle, environmental risk factors, age, and others may play a role in AMD development. However, association of environmental and genetic factors and gene-environment interactions with risk, have been reported to be closely related with the development of AMD [8]. Age is the strongest known risk factor. The older the individual, the higher AMD risk [9–11]. Additionally, a gender has a big impact on AMD development as it was determined that women have a higher risk to develop AMD compared to men [12]. People with blue iris have the higher possibility to develop AMD than people with other iris colors [13]. The meta-analysis of the prospective cohort and cross-sectional studies suggested that darker (brown) iris pigmentation was protective, however, the overall results were not significant [13]. Moreover, ethnicity may influence AMD development. Caucasians are more often diagnosed with AMD than black people. Wong et al. reported a higher prevalence of early and any AMD in Europeans than Asians or Africans as in geographical regions; cases of early and any AMD were less prevalent in Asia than in Europe and North America [11]. Controversial results by different studies have been reported on a risk factor such as sunlight. One study found no association between AMD and sun exposure or related factors except for an association between sunburn prone skin type and geographic atrophy which reached borderline significance [14], while the other study concluded that AMD was probably related to visible radiation, especially blue light [15]. Smoking is another significant and modifiable factor. Many studies have determined the influence of smoking on AMD formation and demonstrated that former and current smokers are inclined to develop AMD at least 5–10 years earlier than nonsmokers [16]. Higher systolic blood pressure, overweight and obesity, and physical exercise duration and frequency are associated with late AMD in women only [17]. The prevalence of AMD is significantly higher in patients with myocardial infarction (MI) than in a simple random sample of the population [18]. It was established that prevalence of early AMD in the random sample was 7.3%, while in MI patients, it was 54.5% ($p < 0.001$). AMD increases more with age in females (3.7 and 10.8% at the age 45–54 and 55–64 years, $p < 0.05$, respectively) while in males, frequency of AMD did not differ significantly between latter age groups (9.9% vs. 11.6%; $p > 0.05$) [18]. Increased intake of fish reduced the risk of AMD, particularly for two or more servings per week. Dietary omega-3 fatty intake was inversely associated with AMD comparing the highest vs. lowest quartile. Reduction of risk for AMD with higher intake of omega-3 fatty acids was seen primarily among subjects with low levels (below median) of linoleic acid intake, an omega-6 fatty acid [19].

Oxidative stress is believed to be a major mediator of the effect of age as mitochondrial oxidation impairment with aging and oxidative damage is widely observed. Oxidative stress and the production of reactive oxygen species seem to play a pivotal role in AMD pathogenesis [20]. The levels of inflammatory markers, such as serum high-sensitivity C-reactive protein, tumor necrosis factor-α receptor 2, interleukin-6, and soluble vascular cell adhesion molecule-1, in blood, were moderately associated to the 20-year cumulative incidence of early AMD independent of age, smoking status, and other factors [21].

More recently, the data from the Age-Related Eye Disease Study showed that cataract surgery is safe in the setting of dry AMD and no accelerate progression to advanced sight threatening forms of AMD were observed [22]. There is a probable relationship between cataracts and the aging process, manifesting in cataract formation with partial nuclear sclerosis and AMD. Some researchers found no link between the cloudy lens and AMD, whereas the others have revealed a relationship between the lens nuclear sclerosis and AMD. West et al. and Klein et al. suggested that nuclear sclerosis of the lens than cortical cloudiness is more often observed in the patients with AMD [23–25]. Progression of AMD in the operated eye due to cataract was more commonly observed than in the patients without the intervention. Moreover, late AMD in the operated eyes developed within 5 years after operation [24].

Levels of vitamin D serum are inversely associated with early, but not advanced, AMD. Consistent use versus non-use of vitamin D from supplements was inversely associated with early AMD only in individuals who did not consume milk daily [26]. Increased blood levels of homocysteine are associated with increased risk of AMD [27].

A whole genome study of the patients with AMD has determined that the complement H factor gene haplotype increases the possibility of developing AMD [28]. Gold B et al. have studied two independent cohorts consisting of 900 patients with AMD and 400 control group persons, and genetic lesions of two complement system factors, i.e., the variants of the genetic factor B (BF) (6p21.3) and the second complement factor (C2) (6p21.3) [29]. The gene of apolipoprotein E (Apo E) was found to be associated with development of AMD. Apo E, which codes the plasma protein participating in the metabolism of cholesterol and other lipids [30], is determined in drusen [31, 32]. The second major locus of the risk of AMD development is linked to genes *HTRA1* and *ARMS2* [33]. In 2013, a genome-wide association study identified seven new loci near genes *COL8A1-FILIP1L, IER3-DDR1, SLC16A8, TGFBR1, RAD51B, ADAMTS9,* and *B3GALTL* [34].

In recent years, the blockage of the neovascularization chain has been considered to inhibit the development of AMD. The vascular endothelial growth factor (VEGF) and the fibroblast growth factor are believed to promote the angiogenesis [35]. Meanwhile, it is inhibited by the pigment epithelial factor, angiostatin, endostatin, and other enzymes. The neovascularization is mainly induced by retinal hypoxia. Tissue ischemia leads to increased secretion of the

VEGF and higher expression of the VEGF R2. Vasodilatation induced by VEGF enhances vascular permeability and protease activity that results in developing and expansion of vascular network of the surrounding tissues and its remodeling [36]. The fragmentation of a basilar membrane and an intracellular connective tissue are essential for the formation of new capillaries. Activated endothelial cells release matrix metalloproteinases which, by degrading the basilar membrane, allow capillaries to grow beneath the retina and between retinal layers, creating favorable conditions for AMD development.

4. Age-related macular degeneration clinics and diagnostics

During the initial stage of AMD, first symptoms of the disease include blurred or fuzzy vision. Patients complain that in Amsler grid of straight horizontal and vertical lines appear wavy, blurred or distorted or boxes in the grid look square and in the different size. Later, in the center of the visual field appears dark area which interferes with vision [37–39]. First symptom of the dry AMD is blurred vision which later would transform into central scotoma, e.g., a black spot in the center of the vision field. This is especially noticeable while reading or looking at objects closely. In the beginning, the disease is asymptomatic and changes in the eye fundus would not cause any complains to the patient. A dry form of AMD usually advances slowly and it takes long months to notice the changes of vision. Sometimes dry form of AMD shifts to the wet form. An exudative AMD is associated with sudden loss of vision, sometimes in a few days' time. Up to 90% of all exudative AMD cases would lead to the total blindness. The Amsler grid test is a simple test which is used at home to check whether lines look wavy or distorted, or areas of the visual field are missing. If any of these changes are detected, the ophthalmologist should be contacted immediately. Examination of retina's central part (the macula) is performed by using the Amsler grid. Each eye is tested separate, and the patient holds the Amsler's grid approximately 40 cm from his eyes and looks to a spot in the middle of a standard grid. It is observed whether there are no wavy or invisible places, and crooked or patchy thickness lines. If a patient sees straight lines, the test is evaluated as negative. Positive test usually is confirmed for patients with the advanced AMD; thus if any complains occur, the ophthalmologist should be contacted and treatment should be started. A detailed anamnesis is needed for an accurate diagnosis of AMD. It would help to identify a cause of a condition and risk factors which may influence the AMD development. An ordinary eye examination starts from an evaluation of eyesight sharpness which abroad is evaluated by using a chart of an Early Treatment Diabetic Retinopathy Study (ETDRS), while in Lithuania—the Snellen chart. ETDRS is an accurate (in case of low visual acuity) with a small error, objective, vigorously scientific method [40]. It is important constantly to check visual acuity for a comparison of previous checkup results. Various diagnostic ophthalmological methods are used to diagnose AMD: perimetry, Amsler's grid testing, functional acuity contrast sensitivity, direct and indirect ophthalmoscopy, scanning laser ophthalmoscopy, color fundus photography with blue and red light filters, fluorescein angiography or with indocyanine green and histological research and electronic biomicroscopy, optical coherent tomography. After performance of color photograph of eye fundus, the progression of AMD should be followed (**Figure 1(a)** (a hard drusen in right eye fundus) and **(b)** (a soft drusen in the left eye fundus)). AMD diagnosis

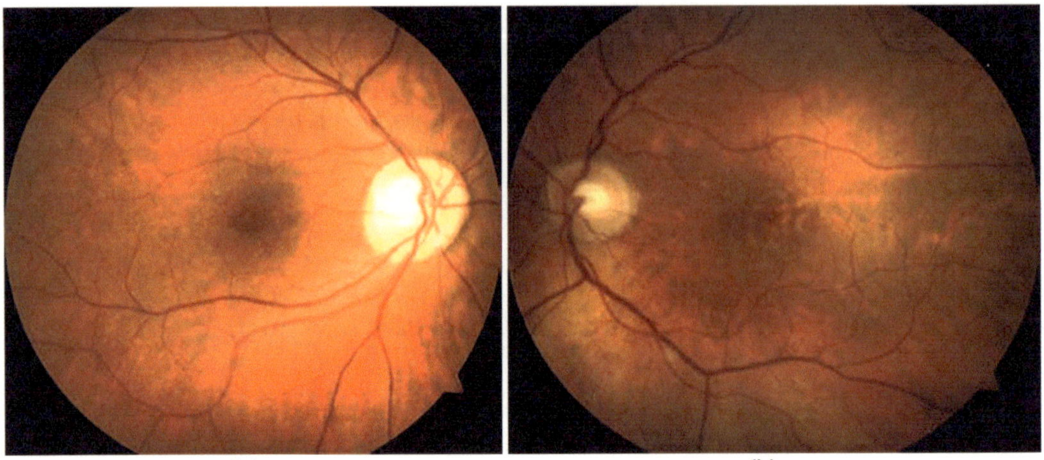

Figure 1. (a) Hard drusen in the right eye fundus and (b) soft drusen in the left eye fundus.

is confirmed after evaluation of clinical symptoms, (and patient's complains) and examination of eye fundus after pupil dilatation with mydriatics (specific changes are checked for in the central retina part). Amsler's grid test and a perimetry (visual field test) are performed to evaluate central eyesight changes. Fluorescein angiography shows a presence of abnormal new blood vessels. The latest method for the confirmation of AMD diagnosis is optical coherent tomography (OCT). This is a non-invasive method, allowing to get good resolution retina photography *in vivo,* to monitor the dynamics of diseases of retina and facilitating diagnostics [41]. OCT provide quantitative and qualitative information on retina condition. Today, OCT is one of additional tools besides eye fundus photography and fluorescence angiography. However, it is step-by-step used instead of previously mentioned methods, especially in monitoring of diseases dynamics during treatment and for determination of retina disease stage [40].

5. Diagnostics

5.1. Impact of metalloproteinase structure, activity, and mutation on activity regulation of matrix metalloproteinases (MMP-2, MMP-3, and MMP-9)

The structure of all MMPs identified is similar (**Figure 1**). The main components of MMP molecule are:

- signal sequence, which is important for MMPs release from cell propeptide, to inactivate a signal sequence of *MMP;*
- catalytic metalloproteinase domain, which include Zn^{2+} ion, essential for enzyme activity;
- axial peptide, which connects catalytic domain with hemopexin domain; and
- hemopexin domain, which determines MMPs possibility to cleave an appropriate substrate [42, 43].

Expression of most MMPs in tissues under normal conditions is low and it is induced when remodeling of extracellular matrix (ECM) is required. Various factors might induce MMPs production: cytokines, growth factors, physical stress, cell-extracellular matrix and cell-cell interaction. Westermarck et al. found that there are four mechanisms of action of matrix metalloproteinases:

1. MMPs may affect cell migration by changing the cells from an adhesive to non-adhesive phenotype and by degrading the ECM;
2. MMPs may alter ECM microenvironment leading to cell proliferation, apoptosis, or morphogenesis;
3. MMPs may modulate the activity of biologically active molecules such as growth factor or growth factor receptors by cleaving them or releasing them from the ECM; and
4. MMPs may alter the balance of protease activity by cleaving the enzymes or their inhibitors [44].

Activation of MMPs expression could be caused by various gene polymorphisms in promoter region, when a binding place of transcription factors or other regulating elements is disrupted. *MMP* polymorphisms can be caused by nucleotide changes within promoter region by insertions, substitutions or microsatellite instability [45]. Around 90% of cases, a single nucleotide polymorphism is determined where one of the basic changes appears in DNA strain [46]. However, several allele polymorphisms can be determined in *MMP* gene promoter regions. Most parts of detected polymorphisms are not biologically active. Only a small part of polymorphisms which changes gene transcription intensity is biologically active; therefore, they may have an impact on genetic predisposition to certain diseases [45]. A common variant in the promoter region of the human matrix metalloproteinase-3 (*MMP-3*) gene with 1 allele having a run of 5 adenines (5A) and the other having 6 adenines (6A) has an impact on gene expression. *MMP-3* gene is located in chromosome 11 11q22.2-11q22.3 region. Insertion of one adenine (A) in -1171 base-pair position of *MMP-3* promoter caused 6 adenines (6A) formation instead of 5 adenines (5A). It was shown that 6A allele has a higher binding affinity to ZBP-89 transcription factor, which decreases promoter transcription activity and certain gene expression [47]. *In vitro* methods showed that 5A allele has a higher activity and effect on gene expression compared to 6A allele [48]. *Ex vivo* method showed that *MMP-3* mRNA and protein activity depends on genotype: 5A/5A shows the highest activity, 5A/6A—the middle activity and the lowest activity shows 6A/6A genotype [47, 48]. A mutation (NCBI SNP identification no. rs2285053) which causes an increase in promoter activity was determined in the *MMP-2* (-735) gene promoter transcription region. *MMP-2* gene is located in 16q13-q21 region. The C to T allelic variation located at nucleotide -735 disrupts the Sp1-binding site in promoter region and significantly leads to a low transcriptional activity; therefore, T allele has a markedly lower promoter activity than the C allele [49]. In addition, another C to T allelic variation located in *MMP-2* at nucleotide -1306 (NCBI SNP identification no. rs243865) disrupts the SP1-binding site of transcription factor in promoter region. It is a similar effect as it happens for *MMP-2* (-735) gene promoter transcription region mutation [50], where promoter loses 50% activity [51]. A transition of C to T at the 1562 base-pair position upstream of the transcription initiation site (-1562 C/T) of *MMP-9* (NCBI SNP identification no. rs3918242) has shown to have an effect on promoter activity. Transition of C nucleotide to T nucleotide causes more difficulties for nucleic protein complex bind to DNA strain in the presence of T allele. It was determined that once C allele mutates to T allele, a promoter activity increases 1.5 times [52]. *MMP-9* gene is located in 20q11.2-q13.1 region. Matrix metalloproteinases are involved in vascular remodeling, and these appear to be active agents degrading extracellular matrix proteins. Their expression in transcription level depends on gene promoter mutations and various transcription factors.

6. Expression of matrix metalloproteinases in human retina and choroid

Bruch's membrane is a pentalaminated extracellular matrix allowing bidirectional diffusion pathways between the retinal pigment epithelium and the choroidal blood supply. Aging is associated with progressive thickening of retina due to deposition of matrix components and membranous debris rich in lipids. A consequence of the aging process is an exponential decline in the hydraulic conductivity of Bruch's membrane [53]. Hemato-retinal barrier might be disrupted only when lesion in Bruch's membrane or in retinal pigment epithelium occurs. Li et al. found that MMP-3, and MMP-2 and -9 were present in human Bruch's membrane, and that the level of the two inactive gelatinases increased with the age of the donor. Regional differences were apparent in the levels of the two gelatinases. The level of MMP-9 remained invariant, while MMP-2 was lower in the macular region than in the periphery [54]. Given that the thickness of Bruch's membrane increases with age and that of choroid decreases, the observed increase in MMP levels is likely to occur mainly in Bruch's membrane. Cultured retinal pigment epithelium (RPE) cells have been reported to synthesize and secrete MMP-1, -2, -3, and -9, and TIMPs as well. The origin of the various MMPs found in Bruch's membrane and choroid remains unknown. The three potential sources are: (1) RPE cells, (2) choroidal cells, and (3) plasma in the choroidal vessels [55, 56].

There are two pathways whereby these enzymes may be incorporated into Bruch's membrane. First, the enzymes may be released from plasma, RPE, and/or choroidal cells and then diffuse into Bruch's membrane. This is certainly a possibility for the smaller molecular weight forms such as MMP-1 (52 kDa), MMP-2 (65 kDa), and MMP-3 (57 kDa), because the molecular weight exclusion limit for Bruch's membrane is approximately 65–75 kDa. Second, the release of MMPs may be coincident with the synthesis of structural components of Bruch's membrane and, therefore, may be incorporated passively into the ECM of Bruch's membrane. Such a pathway would allow an incorporation of higher molecular weight enzymes such as MMP-9 [57].

MMP-1, MMP-2, MMP-3, and MMP-9 expressions are regulated by various ways such as transcription level, activation of latent MMPs, and inhibition of MMP activity by tissue inhibitors of metalloproteinases (TIMPs) [58]. TIMPs are known as natural tissue inhibitors, which regulate active and non-active balance of MMP forms. MMPs are initially expressed in an enzymatically inactive state due to the interaction of a cysteine residue of the pro-domain with the zinc ion of the catalytic site. Only after disruption of this interaction by a mechanism called cysteine switch, which is usually mediated by proteolytic removal of the pro-domain or chemical modification of the cysteine residue, the enzyme becomes proteolytically active. Choroidal neovascularization (CNV) is associated with an upregulation of MMP-9 at the transcriptional level and an activation of pro-MMP-2 by MT1-MMP. This process might be blocked by physiological/natural (TIMP-1 and TIMP-2) and also synthetic inhibitors [59].

MMPs are thought to play a key role during the early phases of choroidal neovascularization. The synthetic inhibitor interacting preferentially with MMP-2, MMP-9, and MT1-MMP (MMP-14) is more efficient comparing to a broad-spectrum synthetic inhibitor in case of choroidal neovascularization. MMPs might have contrary functions—induce or block choroidal neovascularization development [59].

7. Matrix metalloproteinases (MMP-2, -3, and -9) association with age-related macular degeneration

Studies on the morphogenesis of AMD draw attention to the role of MMPs. These studies have confirmed that ECM dysmetabolism plays an important role in the pathogenesis of AMD [60, 61] and metabolism of the ECM is closely regulated by MMPs [62]. The pathogenesis of age-related macular degeneration is mostly focused on MMP-2 and MMP-9, due to their ability to split gelatin *in vitro*.

There are no many studies analyzing MMP-2 influence on AMD development. Some studies analyzed MMP-2 concentration in the blood, some MMP-2 expression, and some analyzed genes' polymorphism in different promoters' regions. To our knowledge, currently there are only two studies analyzing *MMP-2* gene (-1306) C/T polymorphism influence on AMD development [63, 64]. The study done by Seitzman et al. analyzed *MMP-2* (-1306) C/T gene polymorphism in females with AMD, where association between *MMP-2* and early or late AMD in older women was not found [63]. The following study done by Ortak et al. also analyzed genotype distributions and allelic frequencies of *MMP2* (-1306C > T). No significant differences in either genotype distribution or allelic frequencies of *MMP2* (-1306C > T) were found among the patients with dry AMD, wet AMD, and control group [64]. An allele of *MMP-2* rs2287074 was less prevalent in subjects with late AMD than in those with early or no AMD ($p = 0.01$) [63]. The third study also proved that analysis of *MMP-2* (-1306 C/T) gene polymorphism has not revealed any differences in the genotype distribution between patients with early AMD and reference group subjects when analyzed in overall groups, but *MMP-2* gene C/C genotype was more frequent in AMD patients younger than 65 years comparing to AMD group ≥65 years (67.21% vs. 49.37%, $p = 0.039$), and C/T genotype was more frequent in AMD patients ≥65 years comparing to AMD patients <65 years (26.23% vs. 44.3%, $p = 0.033$) [65]. MMP-2 expression in experimental models [66] and in Bruch's membrane-choroid preparations in human donors eyes with AMD diagnosis also were analyzed [67]. Berglin et al. detected low expression of MMP-2 in choroidal neovascularization membrane of mice [66]. In consistent, other scientists group also found a significant reduction in the development of laser-induced CNV in MMP-2 knockout mice [68]. Hussain et al. demonstrated that the total level of active

MMP-2 was significantly reduced in Bruch's membrane-choroid preparations of human donor eyes with AMD [67]. As positive association between MMP-2 expression and choroidal neovascularization was observed, in contrary, a potentially protective role of MMP-2 in dry AMD was suggested. As noted above, estrogen depletion in ovariectomized mice resulted in a loss of MMP-2 expression and subsequent changes associated with dry AMD, such as sub-RPE deposit formation and Bruch's membrane thickening occurred [69]. In others two studies [33, 70], there were no differences in MMP-2 concentration found between AMD and control group. MMP-2 levels in human plasma among healthy individuals, AMD patients, and exudative AMD patients gave a confirmation that the mean concentration of MMP-2 in the early and neovascular AMD was not significantly different from that of the control group [70].

MMP-3 is a key member of the MMPs family and plays a central role in the physiological and pathological events associated with connective tissue metabolism and remodeling [71, 72]. Only few studies have been conducted to clarify if MMP-3 has an influence on retinal vascular remodeling and stiffening, and plays a role in the development of AMD. Literature data concerning MMP-3 effect on AMD are scarce and inconsistent. Some results reveal a possible MMP-3 effect on AMD pathogenesis [73], and at the same time are in conflict with controversial data from the other study assuming that MMP-3 expression did not play a role on AMD development [74]. The study analyzing *MMP-3* gene polymorphism on age-related macular degeneration development in patients with myocardial infarction was carried as well. The study results revealed that *MMP-3* gene polymorphism did not have any predominant effect on the development of AMD in patients with myocardial infarction [75]. German study showed that MMP-3 expression in the retinal pigment epithelium was induced by oxidative stress. It is known that oxidative stress is one of the risk factors for the development of AMD, and it is possible that MMP-3 might affect the development of AMD in this way [73]. Swedish researchers conducted a study where the expression of several MMPs, including MMP-3, was analyzed, but no data suggesting MMP-3 involvement in the development of AMD were found [75].

The studies analyzing an association between MMP-9 and AMD are inconsistent as well. In a few studies, a reduction in MMP-9 was found in choroidal neovascular membranes [76] and in serum [33], while other studies showed an increase in MMP-9 in the aqueous humor [77], plasma [78], and choroidal neovascular membranes [79]. To our knowledge, only one study done by Fiotti et al. revealed the influence of the MMP-9 genotype, which causes greater gene expression on AMD [79]. This study found a relationship between the length of *MMP-9* gene promoter microsatellites and choroidal neovascularization in AMD patients. It has been determined that carriers of one allele with 22 repeats have more than double the risk of AMD. This polymorphism does not cause the disease but increases the MMP-9 expression leading to increased vascular permeability and choroidal neovascularization [80]. No difference between the major AMD risk factors (gender, age, diabetes mellitus, cigarette smoking, and dyslipidemia) and *MMP-9* polymorphism was found. The logistic regression analysis showed that the status of carrier of a microsatellite 22 repeats was the only variable entering into the equation ($p = 0.011$). The only one association was high body mass index value which is linked to a higher risk of developing AMD [80]. The number of cytosine-adenine (CA) sequences in the *MMP-9* gene promoter region was found to determine the transcription activity [45]. Studies with mice mesangial cells have shown that 24 repeats of (CA) sequences in the *MMP-9* gene promoter region result in up to 20 times higher MMP-9 expression compared with 20 repeats of (CA) sequence [81]. Steen et al. suggests that MMP-2 and MMP-9 may be cooperatively involved in the progressive growth of choroidal neovascular membranes in AMD [74]. Lambert et al. demonstrated a significant reduction in the development of laser-induced choroidal neovascularization in MMP-9 knockout mice suggesting that MMP-9 may be important in the pathogenesis of AMD [76], and in Bruch's membrane-choroid preparations from donor eyes, the total level of active MMP-9 was significantly reduced too [67]. Interestingly, a recent study reported that MMP-9 was significantly elevated in the aqueous humor of patients with neovascular AMD [77] and in the plasma in AMD and CNV groups [70]. Zeng et al. showed different results and demonstrated no relationship between the increased levels of circulating MMP-9 and AMD [33]. Chau et al. found opposite results and proved that the mean plasma levels of MMP-2 were not significantly different in the three groups but, the mean plasma MMP-9 levels were significantly higher in AMD and CNV groups compared to that of the control group (265 ± 134, 659 ± 315, and 740 ± 494 ng/mL ($p = 0.008$)) [78]. To our knowledge, there is only one study analyzing the impact of *MMP-2*, *MMP-3*, and *MMP-9* genes polymorphism on the development of early AMD. This study proved that the frequency of the *MMP-2* (-735) C/T and *MMP-3* (-1171) 5A/6A genotypes did not differ significantly between the patients with early AMD and the control group, while the *MMP-9* (-1562) C/C genotype was more frequently detected in patients with AMD than the control group (73.7% vs. 64.6%, $p = 0.048$). The logistic regression analysis showed that the *MMP-9* (-1562) C/C genotype increased the likelihood to develop early AMD (OR = 1.51, 95% CI: 1.01–2.21; $p = 0.046$). After the subdivision into the groups by age, a significant difference only in the frequency of the *MMP-9* (-1562) C/C genotype was found comparing the AMD patients and the control group younger than 65 years (79.7% vs. 66.4%, $p = 0.039$) [65].

8. Conclusions

Age-related macular degeneration is a multifactorial disorder. Alteration of matrix metalloproteinases plays a very important role in AMD pathogenesis, especially in the early phases of choroidal neovascularization. During pathological process, MMP-2, MMP-3, and MMP-9 are present in human Bruch's membrane and RPE at different level and position, and are involved in the inflammatory process. MMP-2, MMP-3, and MMP-9 expressions are regulated by various ways: a transcription, activation of latent MMPs, and inhibition of MMP activity by tissue inhibitors of metalloproteinases. However, knowledge on MMP-2, MMP-3, and MMP-9 action in AMD pathogenesis is still controversial, therefore further research is necessary.

Acknowledgements

Financial support: Lithuanian Science Council (grant no. MIP-10330).

Author details

Rasa Liutkeviciene[1,2]*, Vykintas Liutkevicius[3], Agne Giedraitiene[4], Loresa Kriauciuniene[1,2] and Virginija Asmoniene[5]

*Address all correspondence to: rliutkeviciene@gmail.com

1 Department of Ophthalmology, Medicine Academy, Lithuanian University of Health Sciences, Lithuania

2 Neuroscience Institute, Medicine Academy, Lithuanian University of Health Sciences, Lithuania

3 Department of Otolaryngology, Medicine Academy, Lithuanian University of Health Sciences, Lithuania

4 Institute of Microbiology and Virology, Lithuanian University of Health Sciences, Lithuania

5 Department of Genetics and Molecular Medicine, Medicine Academy, Lithuanian University of Health Sciences, Lithuania

References

[1] Klein R, Peto T, Bird A, Vannewkirk MR. The epidemiology of age-related macular degeneration. American Journal of Ophthalmology. 2004;**137**:486-495

[2] Vingerling JR, Hofman A, Grobbee DE, de Jong PT. Age-related macular degeneration and smoking. The Rotterdam Study. Archives of Ophthalmology 1996;**114**:1193-1196.

[3] De Jong PT. Age-related macular degeneration. The New England Journal of Medicine. 2006;**355**(14):1474-1483

[4] Tomany SC, Wang JJ, Van Leeuwen R, Klein R, Mitchell P, Vingerling JR, et al. Risk factors for incident age-related macular degeneration: Pooled findings from 3 continents. Ophthalmology. 2004;**111**:1280-1287

[5] Friedman DS, O'Colmain BJ, Munoz B, Tomany SC, McCarty C, de Jong PT et al. Prevalence of age-related macular degeneration in the United States. Archives of Ophthalmology 2004;**122**:564-572.

[6] Grizzard SW, Arnett D, Haag SL. Twin study of age-related macular degeneration. Ophthalmic Epidemiology. 2003;**10**:315-322

[7] Zeng R, Wen F, Zhang X, Serum SY. levels of matrix metalloproteinase 2 and matrix metalloproteinase 9 elevated in polypoidal choroidal vasculopathy but not in age-related macular degeneration. Molecular Vision. 2013;**19**:729-736

[8] Hyman LG, Lilienfeld AM, Ferris FL, Fine SL. Senile macular degeneration: A case-control study. American Journal of Epidemiology. 1983;**118**(2):213-227

[9] VanNewkirk M, Nanjan M, Wang J, Mitchell P, Taylor HR, McCarty CA. The prevalence of age-related maculopathy: The visual impairment project. Ophthalmology. 2000; **107**(8):1593-1600

[10] Klein R, Cruickshanks KJ, Nash SD, Krantz EM, Nieto FJ, Huang GH, et al. The prevalence of age-related macular degeneration and associated risk factors. Archives of Ophthalmology. 2010;**128**:750-758

[11] Hyman L, Neborsky R. Risk factors for age-related macular degeneration: An update. Current Opinion in Ophthalmology. 2002;**13**:171-175

[12] Rudnicka AR, Jarrar Z, Wormald R, Cook DG, Fletcher A, Owen CG. Age and gender variations in age-related macular degeneration prevalence in populations of European ancestry: A meta-analysis. Ophthalmology. 2012;**119**(3):571-580

[13] Chakravarthy U, Wong TY, Fletcher A, Piault E, Evans C, Zlateva G, et al. Clinical risk factors for age-related macular degeneration: A systematic review and meta-analysis. BMC Ophthalmology. 2010;**10**:31

[14] Khan JC, Shahid H, Thurlby DA, Bradley M, Clayton DG, Moore AT, et al. Age related macular degeneration and sun exposure, iris colour, and skin sensitivity to sunlight. The British Journal of Ophthalmology. 2006;**90**(1):29-32

[15] Yam JC, Kwok A. Ultraviolet light and ocular diseases. International Ophthalmology. 2014;**34**(2):383-400

[16] Khan JC, Thurlby DA, Shahi H, Clayton DG, Yates JRW. Smoking and age related macular degeneration: The number of pack years of cigarette smoking is a major determinant of risk for both geographic atrophy and choroidal neovascularisation. The British Journal of Ophthalmology. 2006;**90**(1):75-80

[17] Erke MG, Bertelsen G, Peto T, Sjølie AK, Lindekleiv H, Njolstad I. Cardiovascular risk factors associated with age-related macular degeneration: The Tromsø Study. Acta Ophthalmologica. 2014;**92**(7):662-669

[18] Liutkeviciene R, Lesauskaite V, Zaliuniene D, Zaliaduonyte-Peksiene D, Cimbalas A, Jasinskas V, et al. Early age-related macular degeneration in patients with myocardial infarction. Current Eye Research. 2012;**37**(2):94-100

[19] Seddon JM, George S, Rosner B. Cigarette smoking, fish consumption, omega-3 fatty acid intake, and associations with age-related macular degeneration: The US Twin Study of Age-Related Macular Degeneration. Archives of Ophthalmology. 2006;**124**(7): 995-1001

[20] Blasiak J, Petrovski G, Veréb Z, Facskó A, Kaarniranta K. Oxidative stress, hypoxia, and autophagy in the neovascular processes of age-related macular degeneration. BioMed Research International. 2014;**2014**:768026

[21] Klein R, Myers CE, Cruickshanks KJ, Gangnon RE, Danforth LG, Sivakumaran TA, et al. Markers of inflammation, oxidative stress, and endothelial dysfunction and the 20-year cumulative incidence of early age-related macular degeneration: The Beaver Dam Eye Study. JAMA Ophthalmology. 2014;**132**(4):446-455

[22] Chew EY, Sperduto RD, Milton RC, Clemons TE, Gensler GR, Bressler SB, et al. Risk of Advanced Age-Related Macular Degeneration Following Cataract Surgery in the Age-Related Eye Disease Study: AREDS Report 25. Ophthalmology. 2009;**116**(2):297-303

[23] West SK, Rosenthal FS, Bressler NM, Bressler SB, Munoz B, Fine SL, et al. Exposure to sunlight and other risk factors for age-related macular degeneration. Archives of Ophthalmology. 1998;**107**:875-879

[24] Klein BE, Klein R, Lee KE. Incidence of age-related catarct: The Beaver Dam Eye Study. Archives of Ophthalmology. 1998;**116**:219-225

[25] Klein R, Klein BE, Linton KL. Prevalence of age-related maculopathy: The Dam Study Eye Study. Ophthalmology. 1992;**99**:933-943

[26] Parekh N, Chappell RJ, Millen AE, Albert DM, Mares JA. Association between vitamin D and age-related macular degeneration in the Third National Health and Nutrition Examination Survey, 1988 through 1994. Archives of Ophthalmology. 2007;**125**:661-669

[27] Rochtchina E, Wang JJ, Flood VM, Mitchell P. Elevated serum homocysteine, low serum vitamin B12, folate, and age-related macular degeneration: The Blue Mountains Eye Study. American Journal of Ophthalmology. 2007;**143**:344-346

[28] Klein RJ, Zeiss C, Chew EY, Tsai JY, Sackler RS, Haynes C. Complement factor H polymorphism in age-related macular degeneration. Science. 2005;**308**(5720):385-389

[29] Gold B, Meriam JE, Zernant J, Hancox LS, Taiber AJ, Gehrs K, et al. Variation in factor B (BF) and complement 2 (C2) genes is associated with age-related macular degeneration. Nature Genetics. 2006;**38**(4):458-462

[30] Mahley RW, Rall SC Jr. Apolipoprotein E: Far more than a lipid transport protein. Annual Review of Genomics and Human Genetics 2000;**1**:507-537

[31] Dithmar S, Curcio CA, Le NA, Brown S, Grossniklaus HE. Ultrastructural changes in Bruch's membrane of apolipoprotein E-deficient mice. Investigative Ophthalmology & Visual Science. 2000;**41**:2035-2042

[32] Klaver CC, Klifen M, van Duijn CM, Hofman A, Cruts M, Grobbe DE, et al. Genetic association of apolipoprotein E with age-related macular degeneration. American Journal of Human Genetics 1998;**63**(1):200-206.

[33] Akagi-Kurashige Y, Yamashiro K, Gotoh N, Miyake M, Morooka S, Yoshikawa M, et al. MMP20 and ARMS2/HTRA1 are associated with neovascular lesion size in age-related macular degeneration. Ophthalmology. 2015;**122**(11):2295-2302

[34] Fritsche LG, Chen W, Schu M, Yaspan BL, Yu Y, Thorleifsson G, et al. Seven new loci associated with age-related macular degeneration. Nature Genetics. 2013;**45**:433-439

[35] Lee SH, Schloss GJ, Swain JL. Maintenance of vascular integrity in the embryo requires signaling through the fibroblast growth factor receptor. The Journal of Biological Chemistry. 2006;**275**(43):33679-33687

[36] Švagždys S, Lesauskaitė V. Matrikso metalo proteinazės: piktybinių navikų augimo ir plitimo mechanizmai [Matrix metalloproteinases: The mechanisms of invasion and metastatic development of malignant tumours]. Medicinos teorija ir praktika (Medicine Theory and Practice). 2007;**13**(2):132-138

[37] Jager RD, Mieler WF, Miller JW. Age-related macular degeneration. The New England Journal of Medicine. 2008;**358**:2606-2617

[38] Evans JR, Fletcher AE, Wormald RPL. 28,000 Cases of age related macular degeneration causing visual loss in people aged 75 years and above in the United Kingdom may be attributable to smoking. The British Journal of Ophthalmology. 2005;**89**:550-553

[39] Gupta OP, Brown GC, Brown MM. Age-related macular degeneration: The costs to society and the patient. Current Opinion in Ophthalmology. 2007;**18**:201-205

[40] Pece A, Azzolini C, Parodi MB, Bottoni F, Danzi P, Donati S, et al. Consensus on the diagnosis, treatment and follow-up of patients with age-related macular degeneration eligible for ranibizumab. Expert Review of Ophthalmology. 2012;**7**(3):219-225

[41] Almeida IN, Almeida LN, Almeida Sobrinho EF, Gomes BD, Souza Gda S, Rosa AA, et al. Optical coherence tomography and multifocal electroretinography of patients with advanced neovascular age-related macular degeneration before, during, and after treatment with ranibizumab. Arquivos Brasileiros de Oftalmologia. 2015;**78**(2):105-109

[42] Nagase H, Visse R, Murphy G. Structure and function of matrix metalloproteinases and TIMPs. Cardiovascular Research. 2006;**69**(3):562-573

[43] Patterson ML, Atkinson SJ, Knäuper V, Murphy G. Specific collagenolysis by gelatinase A, MMP-2, is determined by the hemopexin domain and not the fibronectin-like domain. FEBS Letters. 2001;**503**(2-3):158-162

[44] Westermarck J, Kähäri VM. Regulation of matrix metalloproteinase expression in tumor invasion. The FASEB Journal. 1999;**13**(8):781-792

[45] Ye S. Polymorphism in matrix metalloproteinase gene promoters: Implication in regulation of gene expression and sus ceptibility of various diseases. Matrix Biology. 2000;**19**:623-629

[46] Ra HJ, Parks WC. Control of matrix metalloproteinase catalytic activity. Matrix Biology. 2007;**26**:587-596

[47] Ye S, Eriksson P, Hamsten A, Kurkinen M, Humphries SE, Henney AM. Progression of coronary atherosclerosis is associated with a common genetic variant of the human stromelysin-1 promoter which results in reduced gene expression. The Journal of Biological Chemistry. 1996;**271**:13055-13060

[48] Medley TL, Kingwell BA, Gatzka CD, Pillay P, Cole TJ. Matrix metalloproteinase-3 genotype contributes to age-related aortic stiffening through modulation of gene and protein expression. Circulation Research. 2003;**92**:1254-1261

[49] Yu C, Zhou Y, Miao X, Xiong P, Tan W, Lin D. Functional haplotypes in the promoter of matrix metalloproteinases-2 predict risk of the occurence and metastasis of esophageal cancer. Cancer Research. 2004;**64**:7622-7628

[50] Vasku V, Vasku A, Tschöplová S, Izakovicová HL, Semrádová V, Vácha J. Genotype association of C(-735)T polymorphism in matrix metalloproteinase 2 gene with G(8002) A endothelin 1 gene with plaque psoriasis. Dermatology. 2002;**204**(4):262-265

[51] Price SJ, Greaves DR, Watkins H. Identification of novel, functional genetic variants in the human matrix metalloproteinases-2 gene: Role of SP1 in allele-specific transcriptional regalation. The Journal of Biological Chemistry. 2001;**276**(10):7549-7558

[52] Zhang B, Henney A, Eriksson P, Hamsten A, Watkins H, Ye S. Genetic variation at the matrix metalloproteinase-9 locus on chromosome 20q12.2-13.1. Human Genetics. 1999;**105**:418-423

[53] Hogan MJ. Role of the retinal pigment epithelium in macular disease. Transactions: American Academy of Ophthalmology and Otolaryngology. 1972;**76**(1):64-80

[54] Li G, Ali A, Hussain G, Limb GA, Marshall J. Age-gependent variation in metalloproteinase activity of isolated human Bruch's memnbrane and choroid. Investigative Ophthalmology & Visual Science. 1999;**11**:2676-2681

[55] Ruiz A, Brett P, Bok D. TIMP-3 is expressed in the human retinal pigment epithelium. Biochemical and Biophysical Research Communications. 1996;**226**:467-474

[56] Della NG, Campochiaro PA, Zack DJ. Localization of TIMP-3 mRNA expression to the retinal pigment epithelium. Investigative Ophthalmology & Visual Science. 1996;**37**:1921-1924

[57] Hussain AA, Starita C, Marshall J. Molecular weight size exclusion limit and diffusional status of aging human Bruch's membrane. [ARVO Abstract]. Investigative Ophthalmology & Visual Science. 1999;**40**(4):S973

[58] Chakraborti S, Mandal M, Das S, Mandal A, Chakraborti T. Regulation of matrix metalloproteinases: An overview. Molecular and Cellular Biochemistry. 2003;**253**(1-2):269-285

[59] Lambert V, Wielockx B, Munaut C, Galopin C, Jost M, Itoh T, et al. MMP-2 and MMP-9 synergize in promoting choroidal neovascularization. The FASEB Journal. 2003;**17**(15): 2290-2292

[60] Chong NH, Keonin J, Luthert PJ, Frennesson CI, Weingeist DM, Wolf RL, et al. Decreased thickness and integrity of the macular elastic layer of Bruch's membrane correspond to the distribution of lesions associated with age-related macular degeneration. The American Journal of Pathology. 2005;**166**:241-251

[61] Spraul CW, Lang GE, Grossniklaus HE, Lang GK. Histologic and morphometric analysis of the choroid, Bruch's membrane, and retinal pigment epithelium in postmortem eyes with age-related macular degeneration and histologic examination of surgically excised choroidal neovascular membranes. Survey of Ophthalmology. 1999;**44**:10-32

[62] Lim CS, Shalhoub J, Gohel MS, Shepherd AC, Davies AH. Matrix metalloproteinases in vascular disease—A potential therapeutic target? Current Vascular Pharmacology. 2010;**8**:75-85

[63] Seitzman RL, Mahajan VB, Mangione C, Cauley JA, Ensrud KE, Stone KL, et al. Estrogen receptor alpha and matrix metalloproteinase 2 polymorphisms and age-related maculopathy in older women. American Journal of Epidemiology. 2008;**167**(10):1217-1225

[64] Ortak H, Demir S, Ateş O, Benli I, Söğüt E, Sahin M. The role of MMP2 (-1306C>T) and TIMP2 (-418 G>C) promoter variants in age-related macular degeneration. Ophthalmic Genetics. 2013;**34**(4):217-222

[65] Liutkeviciene R, Lesauskaite V, Sinkunaite-Marsalkiene G, Zaliuniene D, Zaliaduonyte-Peksiene D, Mizariene V, et al. The role of matrix metalloproteinases polymorphisms in age-related macular degeneration. Ophthalmic Genetics. 2015 Jun;**36**(2):149-155

[66] Berglin L, Sarman S, van der Ploeg I, Steen B, Ming Y, Itohara S, et al. Reduced choroidal neovascular membrane formation in matrix metalloproteinase-2-deficient mice. Investigative Ophthalmology & Visual Science 2003;**44**:403-408.

[67] Hussain AA, Lee Y, Zhang JJ, Marshall J. Disturbed matrix metalloproteinase activity of Bruch's membrane in age-related macular degeneration. Investigative Ophthalmology & Visual Science. 2011;**52**(7):4459-4466

[68] Plantner JJ, Jiang C, Smine A. Increase in interphotoreceptor matrix gelatinase A (MMP-2) associated with age-related macular degeneration. Experimental Eye Research. 1998;**67**: 637-645

[69] Cousins SW, Marin-Castano ME, Espinosa-Heidmann DG, Alexandridou A, Striker L, Elliot S. Female gender, estrogen loss, and sub-RPE deposit formation in aged mice. Investigative Ophthalmology & Visual Science. 2003;**44**:1221-1229

[70] Chau KY, Sivprasad S, Patel N, Donaldson TA, Luthert PJ, Chong NV. Plasma levels of matrix metalloproteinases-2 and -9 in age-related macular degeneration. Journal of Human Hypertension. 2003;**17**(2):119-124

[71] Lesauskaitė V, Šinkūnaitė G, Benetis R, Grabauskas V, Vaskelyte J, Smalinskiene A, et al. MMP-3 gene polymorphism and dilatative pathology of ascending thoracic aorta. Medicina (Kaunas, Lithuania). 2008;**44**:386-391

[72] Samnegard A, Silveira A, Lundman P, Boquist S, Odeberg J, Hulthe J, et al. Serum matrix metalloproteinase-3 concentration is influenced by MMP-3 1612 5A/6A promoter genotype and associated with myocardial infarction. Journal of Internal Medicine. 2005;**258**:411-419

[73] Alge-Priglinger CS, Kreutzer T, Obholzer K, Wolf A, Mempel M, Kernt M, et al. Oxidative stress-mediated induction of MMP-1 and MMP-3 in human RPE cells. Investigative Ophthalmology & Visual Science. 2009;**50**:5495-54503

[74] Steen B, Sejersen S, Berglin L, Seregard S, Kvanta A. Matrix metalloproteinases and metalloproteinase inhibitors in coronial neovascular membranes. Investigative Ophthalmology & Visual Science. 1998;**39**:2194-2200

[75] Liutkevičienė R, Žaliaduonytė-Pekšienė D, Žaliūnienė D, Gustienė O, Jašinskas V, Lesauskaitė V, et al. Does matrix metalloproteinase-3 polymorphism play a role in age-related macular degeneration in patients with myocardial infarction? Medicina. 2012;**48**(8):404-409

[76] Lambert V, Munaut C, Jost M, Noel A, Werb Z, Foidart JM, et al. Matrix metalloproteinase-9 contributes to choroidal neovascularization. The American Journal of Pathology. 2002;**161**(4):1247-1253

[77] Jonas JB, Tao Y, Neumaier M, Findeisen P. Cytokine concentration in aqueous humour of eyes with exudative age-related macular degeneration. Acta Ophthalmologica (Copenh). 2012;**90**:381-388

[78] Chau KY, Sivprasad S, Patel N, Donaldson TA, Luthert PJ, Chong NV. Plasma levels of matrix metalloproteinases-2 and -9 in age-related macular degeneration. Eye (London, England). 2007;**21**(12):1511-1555

[79] Zeng J, Jiang D, Liu X, Zhu X, Tang L. Matrix metalloproteinases expression in choroidal neovascular membranes. Yan Ke Xue Bao. 2004;**20**(3):191-193

[80] Fiotti N, Pedio M, Battaglia Parodi M, Atamura N, Uxa L, et al. MMP-9 microsatellite polymorphism and susceptibility to exudative form of age-related macular degeneration. Genetics in Medicine. 2007;**4**:272-277

[81] Fornoni A, Wang Y, Lenz O, Striker LJ, Striker GE. Association of a decreased number of d(CA) repeats in the matrix metalloproteinase-9 promoter with glomerulosclerosis susceptibility in mice. Journal of the American Society of Nephrology. 2002;**13**:2068-2076

Chapter 5

Retinal Ischemia: MMP-9; Its Relation to Resveratrol, Baicalein, S-allyl L-cysteine and Chi Ju Di Huang Wan

Hsiao-Ming Chao, Wen-Jin Chao and Ing-Ling Chen

Additional information is available at the end of the chapter

http://dx.doi.org/10.5772/intechopen.69525

Abstract

Ischemia has been reported to be related to matrix metalloproteinase-9 (MMP-9) level upregulation. Neovascular glaucoma (NVG) (in proliferative diabetic retinopathy and central/branch retinal vein occlusion) and age-related macular degeneration are known vision-threatening retinal ischemic disorders. In this review, an extensive discussion has been made into how MMP-9 is related to retinal ischemia and what the underlying mechanisms of various traditional Chinese medicine (TCM) compounds and combinations are. High intraocular pressure-induced retinal ischemic changes were characterized by decreased electroretinogram (ERG) b-wave amplitudes, a loss of choline acetyltransferase (ChAT) immunopositive amacrine neurons/processes, increased Müller's vimentin immunoreactivity, and profound retinal ganglion cell (RGC) death. It has also been observed hypoxia inducible factor-1α (HIF-1α), MMP-9 and vascular endothelium growth factor (VEGF) upregulation at the protein/mRNA levels. After ischemia, both the p38 mitogen-activated protein kinases (MAPKs)-stimulated MMP-9 upregulation and HIF-1α-triggered VEGF overexpression might result in neovascularization. Conclusively, baicalein seems to have neuroprotection via antioxidation, antiapoptosis, HO-1 upregulation and HIF-1α, VEGF, and/or MMP-9 downregulation. Furthermore, baicalein inhibition on retinal ischemia-induced MMP-9 upregulation seems to be "partly" associated with its antioxidation. Additionally, retinal ischemia, oxidative stress, and/or kainate excitotoxicity could be protected by resveratrol: "via MMP-9 and inducible nitric oxide synthetase (iNOS) downregulation, and heme oxygenase-1 (HO-1) upregulation," S-allyl L-cysteine (SAC): "through iNOS, HIF-1α, VEGF inhibition and/or MMP-9 downregulation, and antiapoptosis," Chi Ju Di Huang Wan: "by means of antiapoptosis, antioxidation, MMP-9 downregulation and p38 MAPK inhibition."

Keywords: matrix metalloproteinase-9, retinal ischemia, traditional Chinese medicine, hypoxia inducible factor-1α, vascular endothelium growth factor, p38 mitogen-activated protein kinase, baicalein, resveratrol, inducible nitric oxide synthetase, heme oxygenase-1, S-allyl L-cysteine, Chi–Ju–Di–Huang–Wan

1. Introduction

Central retinal artery occlusion (CRAO) [16], primary open angle glaucoma (in urban areas) [24], diabetic retinopathy (type 2 diabetes) [21], and age-related macular degeneration (AMD; age ≥40 of years [17]) is related to retinal ischemia with the incidences of 0.0018, 4, 2.9, and 0.36%, respectively.

Central/branch retinal vein occlusion (CRVO/BRVO) are also associated with retinal ischemia. Retinal or choroidal ischemia can lead to angiogenesis, associated with subretinal fluid and bleeding. Fifteen percent of AMD patients experience profound central vision loss owing to choroidal neovascularization (CNV), namely neovascular AMD (nvAMD) [11]. This explains why nvAMD becomes a leading cause of blindness in the elderly. Vision deterioration further puts patients at a greater danger of falls and possibility of being in need of residential nursing care. There is an eminent necessity for new agents that trigger the self-protective mechanisms and avoid harmful neovascularization.

Oxidative stress in the human retinal pigment epithelium (hRPE) leads to the upregulation of matrix metalloproteinase-9 (MMP-9). Upregulation of MMP-9 can adversely degrade the extracellular matrix and induce irreversible retinal ganglion cell (RGC) death [9]. Brain ischemia has been reported to trigger MMP-9 upregulation [8]. In AMD, plasma MMP-2 and MMP-9 levels have been also indicated to be upregulated [6]. As a consequence, ischemia or oxidative stress may be related to MMP-9 level upregulation. In AMD, plasma MMP-9 concentrations promote neovascularization throughout the early phases of CNV [6]. Previous results have supported that increases in MMP-9, hypoxia inducible factor-1α (HIF-1α), and vascular endothelium growth factor (VEGF) levels in the retina/RGCs directly have a relation with ischemia [5, 13].

In our previous publications, there were active components of traditional Chinese medicine (TCM) that were proved to be antioxidants such as ferulic acid from Chuang Xiong [1, 2]. These include baicalein from Huángqín (*Scutellaria baicalensis*) [13, 3] and S-allyl L-cysteine (SAC) from old garlic [5]. SAC could also act as a kainate antagonist [4]. In addition, Chi Ju Di Huang Wan (CJDHW), a "vision preserved" TCM combination, was demonstrated to protect against retinal ischemia through the attenuation of apoptosis, increase of antioxidative activity, downregulation of MMP-9, and inhibition of p38 mitogen-activated protein kinase (MAPK) [7]. Besides, efficient components of beverages, such as epigallocatechin-3-gallate [18] in green tea and resveratrol [15] in red wine, were also reported to possess protective effect on retinal ganglion cells injured after optic nerve axotomy and retinal ischemia, respectively. This review aimed at evaluating the effects of the following compounds or TCM combinations on retinal ischemia and their relations to MMPs.

Resveratrol has shown to possess strong antioxidant properties. Resveratrol has also been confirmed to provide neuroprotective effects during cerebral ischemia plus reperfusion (I/R), [19], mice retinal I/R [12], and *in vitro* experimental optic neuropathy [14]. However, the effects of resveratrol are not completely highlighted. Therefore, it has been investigated whether and how resveratrol protects against retinal I/R [15].

Baicalein (5,6,7-trihydroxy-2-phenyl-4H-1-benzopyran-4-one) is a natural flavonoid from *Scutellaria baicalensis*. It has been studied whether baicalein can alleviate retinal ischemia using electroretinogram (ERG), immunohistochemistry [vimentin/glial fibrillary acidic protein (GFAP), choline acetyltransferase (ChAT)], TdT-mediated dUTP-digoxigenin Nick and Labeling (TUNEL), and real time PCR (rtPCR) to detect mRNA levels of HIF-1α, VEGF, MMP-9, and/or heme oxygenase-1 (HO-1). In brain ischemia, baicalein inhibited MMP-9 expression. It has also been examined whether and how baicalein can suppress MMP-9 upregulation induced by retinal I/R [3].

Within macrophages and endotheliums, SAC, an organosulfur compound in aged garlic extracts, serves as an antioxidant [10]. It has been investigated whether and how SAC can protect against retinal ischemia. Changes in Thy-1, HIF-1α, VEGF, or MMP-9 levels were also intensively observed [4, 5].

Traditional CJDHW includes *Fructus lycii* (Gou qi zi), *Chrysanthemi flos* (Ju hua), Chi-Ju-Di-Huang-Wan (CJDHW) is a classic herbal formula, traditionally used to stabilize tear film and decrease abnormalities of the corneal epithelium in dry eye patients. *Liu Wei Di Huang Wan, Rehmanniae Radix Preparata* (Shu di huang), *Corni fructus* (Shan zhu yu), *Rhizoma Dioscoreae* (Shan yao), *Poria* (Fu ling), *Cortex Moutan radicis* (Mu dan pi), and *Alismatis Rhizoma* (Ze xie). The active compounds of CJDHW known to have antioxidant properties include Zeaxanthin and Lutein from F. Lycii and C. Flos and Trehalose from R. Radix preparata. It has been evaluated regarding the protective effects and underlying mechanisms of CJDHW against retinal ischemia [7].

2. Body-research methods

In vivo rat retinal ischemia was induced by high intraocular pressure (HIOP) of up to 120 mmHg for 60 min. The mechanism and management were evaluated by ERG b-wave amplitude measurement, immunohistochemistry, and rtPCR.

Resveratrol related to MMP and others: Drug administration (single intravitreous injection of 5 μL) involved either preischemic (15 min before retinal ischemia) or postischemic administration (15 min after retinal ischemia) of resveratrol (0.05, 0.5 nmol) or vehicle (ethanol; control).

Baicalein related to MMP and others: In vitro, an oxidative stress was also established by incubating dissociated retinal cells with 100-μM ascorbate and 5-μM $FeSO_4$ (iron) for 1 h. The rats or the dissociated cells were 15 min pretreated with baicalein [(5 μL invitreous injection (i.v.i.) preischemia: 0.05 or 0.5 nmol; *in vitro* preoxidation: 100 μM)], vehicle (1% ethanol), or trolox (i.v.i.: 5 nmol; *in vitro*: 100 μM or 1 mM). These treatment effects were also evaluated by TUNEL, Western blotting, or *in vitro* dichlorofluorescein assay. In addition, the rtPCR assessed the retinal mRNA expression of HIF-1α, MMP-9, VEGF, and HO-1. The other *in vitro* methods for hRPE subjected to H_2O_2 (500 μM)-induced oxidative stress included lactate dehydrogenase or enzyme-linked immunosorbent assay to measure cell viability or the levels of VEGF/MMP-9, respectively.

S-allyl L-cysteine related to MMP and others: In vivo excitotoxicity or *in vitro* oxidative stress was also induced by 100 μM kainate injected into a Wistar rat's vitreous for 1 day or 24 h H_2O_2 (500 μM) incubation of RGC-5 cell line. The management and mechanisms of 100 μM SAC (5 μL intravitreous injection or incubation) and/or the kainate receptor antagonist 100 μM CNQX (5 μL intravitreous injection or incubation) applied 15 min preexcitotoxocity/preischemia/preoxidative stress were evaluated by histopathology (TUNEL, fluorogold retrograde labeled RGCs), and various biochemical approaches [inducible nitric oxide synthetase (iNOS), HIF-1α, VEGF and/or MMP-9 mRNA/protein levels].

Chi Ju Di Huang Wan related to MMP and others: The effects of CJDHW were studied by (i) rtPCR for retinal Thy-1 and MMP-9 mRNA levels; (ii) Western blotting for retinal B-cell lymphoma 2 (Bcl-2), HO-1, P-p38 MAPK and MMP-9 protein levels; (iii) Hematoxylin and haematoxylin and eosin (HE) staining; (iv) fluorogold retrograde labeling; and (v) TUNEL apoptosis assay.

A daily oral intake of 3 mL of water (vehicle; Group 2) or CJDHW (2.8 or 4.2 g/kg/day; CJDHW2.8 or CJDHW4.2; Group 3 or 4) was given for 7 consecutive days preischemia or postischemia. In Group 5, 4 μL of 0.5 mM SB203580 (p38 MAPK inhibitor) was intravitreously injected to the ischemic eye (15 min preischemia). The control rats received a sham procedure (Group 1).

3. Conclusion: key results

The role of MMP-9 in a TCM compound or the TCM combination: An invention of a new small-molecule medicine will run through considerable tedious and prolonged processes. These include the selection of a single compound, animal safety study, investigational new drug, preclinical trial, clinical trials, and new drug application. Launching a new medicine might take 10–15 years and cost billions of US dollars. The institutional review board would be somehow strict to the investigators or the pharmaceutical companies when they were involved in implementing their clinical trials.

Artemisinin, one effective compound against malaria, was first isolated from the TCM, Qinghao, and tested in the 1970s in China [22]. Thrillingly, the discovery of artemisinin that awarded Professor Youyou Tu, the first Chinese Nobel Winner of Medicine in 2016 has pushed the era of traditional medicine come around [23]. There are many intractable disorders, such as the ischemia-related vision-threatening eye diseases, namely nvAMD, branch retinal artery occlusion (BRAO)/BRVO, CRAO/CRVO, proliferative diabetic retinopathy (PDR), diabetic macular edema (DME), NVG, or choroidal melanoma as described previously. It is clear that the traditional medicine could be an alternative way, which might be able to be complementary to the modern medicine. With the evidence described above and discussion as follows (**Figure 1**), we hopefully could find a way out to manage with the defined retinal ischemia-associated vision-threatening ocular disorders.

The HIOP-induced retinal ischemic changes were characterized by a decrease in ERG b-wave amplitudes, a loss of choline acetyltransferase immunopositive amacrine cell bodies/neuronal

http://dx.doi.org/10.5772/intechopen.69525

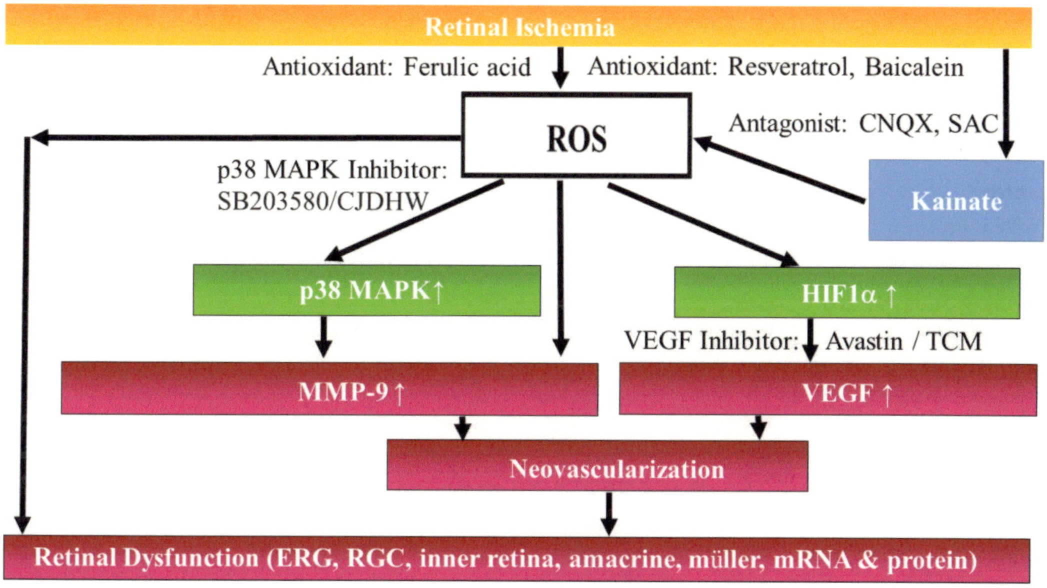

Figure 1. MMP-9 has been reported to play an important role in the retinal ischemia/excitotoxicity/oxidative stress [9, 11–15, 17]. Excitotoxicity and reactive oxygen species (ROS), such as $\cdot O_2$-, H_2O_2 and $\cdot OH$, are widely accepted to be provided through the Fenton reaction in alive cells. The HIOP-induced retinal ischemic changes were characterized by a decrease in ERG b-wave amplitudes, a loss of choline acetyltransferase immunopositive amacrine cell bodies/neuronal processes, an increase in vimentin immunoreactivity, a Müller cell marker and tremendous death of retinal ganglion cells. It has been also observed the upregulation of HIF-1α, MMP-9 and VEGF at the protein/mRNA levels. Both the p38 MAPK-stimulated MMP-9 upregulation and HIF-1α-triggered VEGF overexpression would result in neovascularization. Neovascular glaucoma (in PDR, CRVO/BRVO) and nvAMD are known to be troublesome vision-threatening retinal ischemia-realted ocular disorders. A combination of single compounds or TCM combinations [24] might produce combined drug effects to the commercial agents due to their different treatment mechanisms with less complications. As described previously [9, 11–15, 17], baicalein seems to have protective effect via antioxidation, antiapoptosis, HO-1upregulation and downregulation of HIF-1α, VEGF, and/or MMP-9. Furthermore, the underlying mechanism of the baicalein inhibition on retinal ischemia-induced upregulated MMP-9 level seems to be only ''in part'' associated with its anti-oxidative effect [13]. In addition, retinal ischemia, oxidative stress and/or kainate excitotoxicity could be protected by resveratrol: "via downregulation of MMP-9 and iNOS as well as upregulation of HO-1"; SAC: "through an inhibition of iNOS, HIF-1α, VEGF and/or MMP-9 upregulation as well as apoptosis"; CJDHW: "by means of anti-apoptosis, anti-oxidation, MMP-9 downregulation and p38 MAPK inhibition". Abbreviations: proliferative diabetic retinopathy, PDR; central/branch retinal vein occlusion, CRVO/BRVO; neovascular age related macular degeneration, nvAMD; traditional Chinese medicine, TCM; hypoxia inducible factor-1α, HIF-1α; vascular endothelium factor, VEGF; matrix metalloproteinase-9, MMP-9; inducible nitric oxide synthetase, iNOS; heme oxygenase-1, HO-1; S-allyl L-cysteine, SAC; Chi Ju Di Huang Wan, CJDHW; mitogen-activated protein kinase, MAPK.

processes, and an increase in vimentin immunoreactivity, a Müller cell marker. It has also been observed the upregulation of MMP-9 at the protein/mRNA level.

Resveratrol related to MMP and others: It has also been demonstrated the upregulation of HO-1, and iNOS, as well as the downregulation of Thy-1, at the protein/mRNA level. The ischemic detrimental effects were concentration-dependent (weaker effect at 0.05 nmol) and/or significantly (at 0.5 nmol) altered when resveratrol was applied 15 min before or after retina ischemia. Conclusively, this study supports the hypothesis that resveratrol may be able to protect the retina against ischemia by downregulating MMP-9 and iNOS, and upregulating HO-1.

Baicalein related to MMP and others: The retinal ischemic changes also included Bcl-2 protein linked to an increased apoptotic cells, and changes in the HIF-1α, VEGF, and HO-1 mRNA levels; in hRPEs, H_2O_2 (500 μM) induced oxidative stress was associated with the upregulated VEGF and MMP-9 protein levels. Notably, the ischemic or oxidative injures were concentration-dependent and/or significantly (0.05 nmol and/or 0.5 nmol; 25 and/or 50 μM) altered when baicalein was applied 15 min before retinal ischemia or H_2O_2 (500 μM). In retinal cells or hRPEs subjected to ascorbate/iron or H_2O_2 (500 μM), there was an increased ROS, which was significantly attenuated by 100-μM baicalein and trolox (100 μM or 1mM) or 50/25 μM baicalein which downregulated the VEGF and MMP-9 protein overexpression. Furthermore, the underlying mechanism of the baicalein inhibition on retinal ischemia-induced upregulated MMP-9 level seems to be only "in part" associated with its antioxidative effect [9].

SAC related to MMP and others: Retinal excitotoxic/ischemic changes were also identified by fluorogold retrograde labeled RGCs, and increases in RGC layer apoptotic cells. Upregulated mRNA levels of iNOS, HIF-1α, and/or VEGF were also detected in the retina subjected to kainate excitoxicity or HIOP. The increased HIF-1α and VEGF protein levels were also seen in RGC-5 cells subjected to defined oxidative stress. Importantly, the excitotoxicity/ischemia/oxidative stress-induced alterations were significantly blunted when kainate receptor antagonist 100 μM CNQX and/or SAC (5 μL intravitreous injection or incubation) was applied 15 minutes before ischemia, oxidative stress or excitotoxicity. Conclusively, SAC would seem to protect against retinal ischemia/oxidative stress/kainate excitotoxicity via an inhibition of iNOS, HIF-1α, VEGF and/or MMP-9 upregulation as well as a modulation of glial activation and apoptosis.

CJDHW related to MMP and others: The ischemia-induced changes (Group 2) were significantly modulated by preischemic treatment with CJDHW (Group 4) on I/R day 7. These modulations included (Group 2 *vs.* 4) increased ERG b-wave amplitudes, inner retinal thickness, ChAT immunolabeling amscrines, and RGCs. They also showed decreased vimentin/GFAP immunolabeling Müllers and RGC layer apoptotic cells. Moreover, increased Thy-1 and decreased MMP-9 mRNA (mean: 4.44 *vs.* 1.13) levels were found, respectively. Furthermore, the Bcl-2 protein level increased while the HO-1, P-p38 MAPK (mean: 1.12 *vs.* 0.57) and MMP-9 levels (mean: 0.70 *vs.* 0.39) were decreased. The ischemia-associated increases in P-p38 and MMP-9 protein levels (mean) were also attenuated by 0.5 mM SB203580 (P-p38 MAPK: 1.12 *vs.* 0.18; MMP-9: 0.70 *vs.* 0.21). This was also the case with the MMP-9 enzyme activity (Group 2 *vs.* 4 *vs.* 5: 5.03 *vs.* 1.59 *vs.* 1.35). Conclusively, CJDHW prevented retinal ischemia through antiapoptosis, antioxidation, MMP-9 downregulation, and p38 MAPK inhibition.

A combination of single compounds or TCM combinations [20] might create synergistic pharmaceutical effects to the modern medicine owing to their various therapeutic mechanisms with less unwanted drug effects. Whether the traditional medicine is ready to be complementary to the modern medicine, it is will be clear if the era of Ethnopharmacology would be ready, is not it.

Author details

Hsiao-Ming Chao[1,2,3]*, Wen-Jin Chao[4] and Ing-Ling Chen[5]

*Address all correspondence to: hsiaoming.chao@gmail.com

1 Department of Ophthalmology, Cheng Hsin General Hospital, Taipei, Taiwan

2 Institute of Pharmacology, School of Medicine, National Yang-Ming University, Taipei, Taiwan

3 Department of Chinese Medicine, School of Chinese Medicine, China Medical University, Taichung, Taiwan

4 Department of Biology, University of British Columbia, Vancouver, British Columbia, Canada

5 Department of Medicine, Rush University Medical Center, Chicago, Illinois, USA

References

[1] Chao HM, Lin DE, Chang Y, Hsu WM, Lee SM, Lee FL, Chi CW, Pan WH, Liu TY, Lui WY, Ho LT, Kuo CD, Chan CC, Chao FP. Ferulic acid, but not tetramethylpyrazine, significantly attenuates retinal ischemia/reperfusion-induced alterations by acting as a hydroxyl radical scavenger. Journal of Ocular Pharmacology and Therapeutics. 2008;**24**(5):461-72

[2] Chao HM, Chen YH, Liu JH, Lee SM, Lee FL, Chang Y, Yeh PH, Pan WH, Chi CW, Liu TY, Lui WY, Ho LT, Kuo CD, Lin DE, Chan CC, Yang DM, Lin AM, Chao FP. Iron-generated hydroxyl radicals kill retinal cells in vivo: Effect of ferulic acid. Human & Experimental Toxicology. 2008;**27**(4):327-339

[3] Chao HM, Chuang MJ, Liu JH, Liu XQ, Ho LK, Pan WH, Zhang XM, Liu CM, Tsai SK, Kong CW, Lee SD, Chen MM, Chao FP. Baicalein protects against retinal ischemia by antioxidation, antiapoptosis, downregulation of HIF-1α, VEGF, and MMP-9 and upregulation of HO-1. Journal of Ocular Pharmacology and Therapeutics. 2013;**29**(6):539-549

[4] Chao HM, Chen IL, Liu JH. S-allyl L-cysteine protects the retina against kainate excitotoxicity in the rat. American Journal of Chinese Medicine. 2014;**42**(3):693-708

[5] Chen YQ, Pan WH, Liu JH, Chen MM, Liu CM, Yeh MY, Tsai SK, Young MS, Zhang XM, Chao HM. The effects and underlying mechanisms of S-allyl l-cysteine treatment of the retina after ischemia/reperfusion. Journal of Ocular Pharmacology and Therapeutics. 2012;**28**(2):110-117

[6] Chau KY, Sivaprasad S, Patel N, Donaldson TA, Luthert PJ, Chong NV. Plasma levels of matrix metalloproteinase-2 and 9 (MMP-2 and MMP-9) in age-related macular degeneration. Eye. 2008;**22**:855-859

[7] Cheng JM, Liu XQ, Liu JH, Pan WHT, Zhang XM, Hu L and Chao HM. Chi Ju Di Huang Wan protects rats against retinal ischemia by down regulating matrix metalloproteinase 9 and inhibiting p38 mitogen activated protein kinase. Chinese Medicine. 2016;**11**:39-54

[8] Gao D, Zhang X, Jiang X, Peng Y, Huang W, Cheng G, Song L. Resveratrol reduces the elevated level of MMP-9 induced by cerebral ischemia reperfusion in mice. Life Sciences. 2006;**78**:2564-2570

[9] Guo L, Moss SE, Alexander RA, Ali RR, Fitzke FW, Cordeiro MF. Retinal ganglion cell apoptosis in glaucoma is related to intraocular pressure and IOP-induced effects on extracellular matrix. Investigative ophthalmology & visual science. 2005;**46**:175-182

[10] Kim KM, Chun SB, Koo MS, Choi WJ, Kim TW, Kwon YG, Chung HT, Biliar TR, Kim YM. Differential regulation of NO availability from macrophages and endothelial cells by the garlic component S-allyl L-cysteine. Free Radical Biology and Medicine. 2001;**30**: 747-756

[11] Klein R, Klein BE, Linton KL. Prevalence of age related maculopathy. Beaver Dam Eye Study. Ophthalmology. 1992;**99**:933-943

[12] Li C, Wang L, Huang K, Zheng L. Endoplasmic reticulum stress in retinal vascular degeneration: protective role of resveratrol. Investigative ophthalmology & visual science. 2012;**53**:3241-3249

[13] Liu JH, Wann H, Chen MM, Pan WH, Chen YC, Liu CM, Yeh MY, Tsai SK, Young MS, Chuang HY, Chao FP, Chao HM. Baicalein significantly protects human retinal pigment epithelium cells against H_2O_2-induced oxidative stress by scavenging reactive oxygen species and downregulating the expression of matrix metalloproteinase-9 and vascular endothelial growth factor. Journal of Ocular Pharmacology and Therapeutics. 2010;**26**(5):421-429

[14] Liu Q, Ju WK, Crowston JG, Xie F, Perry G, Smith MA, Lindsey JD, Weinreb RN. Oxidative stress is an early event in hydrostatic pressure induced retinal ganglion cell damage. Investigative Ophthalmology & Visual Science. 2007;**48**:4580-4589

[15] Liu XQ, Wu BJ, Pan WH, Zhang XM, Liu JH, Chen MM, Chao FP, Chao HM. Resveratrol mitigates rat retinal ischemic injury: roles of MMP-9, iNOS, and HO-1. Journal of Ocular Pharmacology and Therapeutics. 2013;**29**(1):33-40

[16] Park SJ, Choi NK, Seo KH, Park KH, Woo SJ. Nationwide incidence of clinically diagnosed central retinal artery occlusion in Korea 2008 to 2011. Ophthalmology. 2014;**121**(10):1933-1938

[17] Park SJ, Kwon KE, Choi NK, Park KH, Woo SJ. Prevalence and incidence of exudative age-related macular degeneration in South Korea: A nationwide population-based study. Ophthalmology. 2015;**122**(10):2063-2070

[18] Peng PH, Chiou LF, Chao HM, Lin S, Chen CF, Liu JH, Ko ML. Effects of epigallocatechin-3-gallate on rat retinal ganglion cells after optic nerve axotomy. Experimental Eye Research. 2010;**90**(4):528-34

[19] Shin JA, Lee H, Lim YK, Koh Y, Choi JH, Park EM. Therapeutic effects of resveratrol during acute periods following experimental ischemic stroke. Journal of Neuroimmunology. 2010;**227**:93-100

[20] Tan SQ, Geng X, Liu JH, Pan WHT, Wang LX, Liu HK, Hu L, Chao HM. Xue-Fu-Zhu-Yu Decoction protects rats against retinal ischemia by downregulation of HIF-1α and VEGF via inhibition of RBP2 and PKM2. BMC. Complementary and Alternative Medicine. 2017; In minor revision (potentially accepted in May 30th 2017).

[21] Thomas RL, Dunstan FD, Luzio SD, Chowdhury SR, North RV, Hale SL, Gibbins RL, Owens DR. Prevalence of diabetic retinopathy within a national diabetic retinopathy screening service. British Journal of Ophthalmology. 2015;**99**(1):64-68

[22] Tu Y. The discovery of artemisinin (qinghaosu) and gifts from Chinese medicine. Nature Medicine. 2011;**17**(10):1217-1220

[23] Tu Y. Artemisinin-A Gift from traditional chinese medicine to the world (Nobel lecture). Angewandte Chemie International Edition in English. 2016;**55**(35):10210-10226

[24] Zhao Y, Fu JL, Li YL, Li P, Lou FL. Epidemiology and clinical characteristics of patients with glaucoma: an analysis of hospital data between 2003 and 2012. Indian Journal of Ophthalmology. 2015;**63**(11):825-31

Section 4

Matrix Metalloproteinases and Skin Diseases

Chapter 6

Skin Ageing and Cancer

Guolong Zhang, Peiru Wang and Xiuli Wang

Additional information is available at the end of the chapter

http://dx.doi.org/10.5772/intechopen.70266

Abstract

Human matrix metalloproteinases (MMPs) belong to the M10 family of the MA clan of endopeptidases. They are ubiquitarian enzymes, structurally characterized by an active site where a Zn^{2+} atom, coordinated by three histidines, plays the catalytic role, assisted by a glutamic acid as a general base. Based on their structure and substrate specificity, they can be categorized into five main subgroups, namely (1) collagenases (MMP-1, MMP-8 and MMP-13); (2) gelatinases (MMP-2 and MMP-9); (3) stromelysins (MMP-3, MMP-10 and MMP-11); (4) matrilysins (MMP-7 and MMP-26) and (5) membrane-type (MT) MMPs (MMP-14, MMP-15, MMP-16, MMP-17, MMP-24 and MMP-25). MMPs can act on extracellular matrix (ECM) and non-ECM components affecting degradation and modulation of the ECM, growth-factor activation and cell-cell and cell-matrix signalling. In skin, MMPs are secreted by different cell types such as fibroblasts, keratinocytes, macrophages, endothelial cells, mast cells, and eosinophils. This chapter reviews the role of MMPs in maintaining skin homeostasis, skin ageing and skin cancer.

Keywords: MMP, skin ageing, photoageing, cutaneous melanoma, cutaneous squamous cell carcinoma, basal cell carcinoma

1. Introduction

Human skin is the largest organ in the human body. The primary function of the skin is to provide a protective barrier against environmental insults, such as heat, solar ultraviolet (UV) irradiation, infection, injury and water loss. The skin is composed of two layers: the epidermis and the dermis [1]. The epidermis is primarily composed of keratinocytes, which produce keratins, intermediate filaments that provide mechanical stability. The dermis is largely composed of dense collagen-rich extracellular matrix. Dermal collagen represents by far the most abundant ECM protein and constitutes the bulk of skin (90% dry weight) [2]. Dermal ECM is essentially responsible for the skin's tensile strength and mechanical properties. In human skin dermis, collagen-rich ECM is synthesized, organized and maintained by dermal fibroblasts [3]. Matrix metalloproteinases (MMPs) are a family of zinc-dependent endopeptidases, which are involved in remodelling of connect tissue of many organs, including the skin [4]. More than 24 MMPs have been identified in human beings, most of which consist of multidomains [5]. MMPs activity is regulated at multiple levels: gene expression, zymogens activation and inhibition by specific inhibitors [4]. In skin, MMPs are produced by several different types of cells such as fibroblasts, keratinocytes, macrophages, endothelial cells, mast cells and eosinophils [6]. MMPs play an important role in maintaining skin homeostasis and various pathophysiological conditions, such as skin ageing, wound healing and skin cancer. The aim of this chapter is to provide a concise overview of the research progress on MMPs in skin ageing and skin cancer.

2. MMPs in skin development and cutaneous wound healing

The active and continuous changes in cell-cell adhesion, cell migration, cell proliferation, apoptosis and remodelling that are required for normal skin development involve MMP gene expression and activation of pro-MMPs. Degradation of dermal ECM is required for epidermal expansion and appendage development during embryogenesis and for the cyclic growth of hair follicles in adult skin. Starting from the third month of gestation, immunostaining for MMP-1 has been detected in basal epidermal keratinocytes and dermal fibroblasts, as well as in cells in and around developing hair follicles [7]. As the development proceeds, the amount of MMP-1 protein decreases, and in adult human skin, MMP-1 is not expressed in intact human epidermis, whereas occasional fibroblast-like cells in the reticular dermis express the mRNA and protein [8]. Matrilysin has been detected in epidermal layers of fetal skin and in cells of early appendageal buds [9]. As skin development continues, matrilysin disappears from epidermal keratinocytes and then expresses in outer root sheath of hair follicles as well as secretory portion of the eccrine glands. Immunostaining for MMP-9 is detected in mesenchymal cells of upper dermis in fetal skin [10], whereas in adult skin, MMP-9 mRNA is detected in the lower epidermis [10]. MMP-2 is constitutively expressed by dermal fibroblasts and occasional basal keratinocytes in normal adult skin [10]. MMP-3 and MMP-10 mRNAs are not expressed in normal intact epidermis or dermis [11], but are occasionally detected in normal hair follicles [6]. MMP-14 expression in fibroblasts plays a crucial role in collagen remodelling in adult skin and largely contributes to dermal homeostasis underlying its pathogenic role in fibrotic skin disease [12]. MMP-21 were present in inflammatory or stromal cells in ageing mice while dysplastic keratinocytes and invasive cancer were negative, suggesting that MMP-21 does not associate with invasion of squamous cell carcinoma (SCC) but may be involved in keratinocyte differentiation [13].

The hair cycle is an intrinsic and cyclic system of regenerating tissue, which is composed of the anagen (phases of rapid growth; 1–3 weeks), catagen (phases of apoptosis-driven regression; ~2 days) and telogen (phases of relative quiescence; ~2 weeks) phases [14]. The hair cycle is considered to be a process of tissue regeneration associated with ECM degradation and remodelling [15]. Increasing evidence demonstrates that MMPs have been suggested to be associated with the hair cycle in vitro and in vivo. Yamazaki et al. reported that MMP-2 was expressed strongly in anagen tissue and slightly in telogen tissue, and topical application of 1% minoxidil sulphate to the anterior dorsal skin of rats in telogen stimulated hair growth and increased the mRNA expressions of hepatocyte growth factor (HGF) and MMP-2 [16]. After stimulation with epidermal growth factor (EGF), tumour necrosis factor-alpha (TNF-α) or interleukin-1 alpha (IL-1α), MMP-9 production was strongly increased in human hair follicles cultured in vitro. Using immunohistochemistry, MMP-9 was detected in the lower part of the inner root sheath (Henle's layer) of normal human anagen hair follicles [17]. These findings suggest that MMP-2 strongly expressed in anagen and may act as hair growth regulatory molecules, whereas the mechanism of the association is largely unknown. Hou et al. further confirmed that MMP-2 and MMP-9 may serve as an important role in the hair growth cycle. The different expressions of MMP-2 and MMP-9 in different stages of hair cycle significantly influenced the collagenase IV expression, which in turn plays an important role in regulating hair cycle by inducing vascular endothelial growth factor (VEGF), insulin-like growth factor (IGF)-1 and transforming growth factor β (TGF-β) expression [15, 18]. So far, there have been no reports of other MMPs associated with hair cycle.

Moreover, there is increasing evidence that MMPs play a crucial role in cutaneous wound healing. MMP-1 expression occurs as a rapid response to wounding and is exclusively expressed in basal keratinocytes at the migrating epithelial front in wounds without basement membrane [19]. Initial expression of MMP-1 is dependent on $\alpha 2\beta 1$ integrin, whereas sustained expression of MMP1 involves cross-talk between the $\alpha 2\beta 1$ integrin and the EGF receptor [20]. Expression of MMP-1 can also be modulated by numerous proinflammatory mediators such as interleukin-1 and TGF-α [21]. Activity of both MMP-2 and MMP-9 can be detected in wound fluids of human mucosal epithelium, suggesting a role for these MMPs in wound healing [22]. Addition of exogenous MMP-2 to primary human nasal epithelial cultures promotes wound closure, which supported the idea that MMP-2 might has a role in wound healing [23]. In mice, expression of MMP-9 is observed at the leading edges during wound closure. MMP-9 knock-out mice display delayed wound closure, suggesting a role for MMP-9 in keratinocyte migration [24]. As is well known, angiogenesis is an important step during wound healing. Both MMP-2 and MMP-9 play a role in physiologic angiogenesis, suggesting that MMP-2 and MMP-9 can have a critical role in this process. MMP-3 and MMP-10 have a differential pattern of expression, with MMP-3 being expressed by a proliferating population adjacent to the wound edge, whereas MMP-10 is expressed at the leading edge, where it colocalizes with MMP-1. Keratinocytes expressing MMP-3 are in contact with an intact basement membrane, while MMP-10 expression is induced in keratinocytes migrating on type I collagen [11]. MMP-10 expression seems to be regulated by cytokines such as EGF, TGF-β1 and TNF-α [25]. MT1-MMP localizes at the migrating front in migrating keratinocytes, accompanied by pro-MMP-2 activation, a coordinated process involving two molecules of MT1-MMP and also TIMP-2 [26]. MT1-MMP may be involved in the regulation of epithelial cell proliferation after tissue injury through a mechanism involving keratinocyte growth factor (KGF) receptor expression [27]. In-vitro data show that MT1-MMP can cleave syndecan-1, CD44 and laminin-332, accelerating migration of different epithelial cells [28, 29]. MMP-8, which is mainly expressed by neutrophils, was discovered to be the most abundant collagenase in human cutaneous excisional wounds [30]. In wound healing, MMP-8 can compensate for loss of MMP-13 expression in MMP-13-defficient mice, and MMP-8 knockout mice demonstrate a significant delay in wound healing [31]. MMP-12 is produced by macrophages in the wound area in acute murine excisional wounds, being detected mainly around the blood vessels [32]. These results, together with more recent data showing that MMP-12 can generate angiostatin, suggest a potential role of MMP-12 in angiogenesis [33]. MMP-13 is expressed in mice at the leading edge of cutaneous wounds. Data obtained with MMP-13 knockout mice suggest that MMP-13 plays a role in keratinocyte migration, angiogenesis and contraction in wound healing [34]. Metalloproteinase-19 has been detected in proliferating epithelium, fibroblasts, capillary endothelial cells and also macrophages in skin wounds [35]. Overexpression of MMP-19 in a epidermal keratinocyte cell line in vitro increased cellular proliferation, migration and adhesion to type I collagen through a mechanism involving the insulin-like growth factor (IGF)-binding protein-3 and the IGF-I receptor [36]. MMP-26, the smallest MMP, has been shown to be expressed during re-epithelialization in cutaneous wound healing. Its expression has been detected in migrating keratinocytes at the wound edge [37]. MMP-28 seems to be expressed by proliferating keratinocytes distal from the wound edge. It is suggested that MMP-28 may be needed to restructure the basement membrane or to degrade cellular adhesion proteins between keratinocytes in order to supply new cells for the migrating front [38].

3. MMPs in skin ageing

3.1. Ageing of human skin

Ageing of human skin can be caused by passage of time (intrinsic or chronological ageing) or environmental factors such as light, heat, cold, etc. (extrinsic ageing or photoageing). Intrinsic skin ageing is a slow, spontaneous, progressive, cumulative and degradative process represents as both epidermal and dermal atrophy. Clinical changes of intrinsic skin ageing show only finely wrinkled at old age (>70 years). The histopathology manifests epidermal atrophy, flattening of the rete ridges and dermal ECM reduction [3].

Chronic exposition to solar UV irradiation is the major extrinsic factor accelerates skin ageing. Usually, photoageing also means extrinsic skin ageing. Clinically, photoageing is recognizable by fine and coarse wrinkles, blotchy dyspigmentation, telangiectasia, sallowness, increased fragility and rough skin texture [39]. Histologically, the epidermal becomes thick during photoageing; the dermal connective tissue is composed of damaged and disorganized collagen fibrils and massive accumulation of aberrant elastic material, referred to as "solar elastosis" [3]. The action spectrum for UV-induced skin damage is divided into (320–400 nm) and UV-B (290–320 nm). The 95% of the UV radiation reaching the Earth's surface is UVA, which is only slightly affected by ozone levels. Although, the amount of UVB reaching the earth's surface is lesser than that of UVA, its intensity is high enough to induce photoageing and skin cancer [39]. In past decades, several studies reported that solar UV irradiation induce different kinds of MMPs leading to photoageing.

Dermal ECM in particular the collagen and elastic fibres changes, is the major alteration in both intrinsic ageing and photoageing. Imbalance of collagen synthesis and breakdown causes alternations of dermal collagen. In both extrinsic and intrinsic ageing, elevated levels and activities of cutaneous MMPs have been demonstrated [3, 40].

Type I collagen is the most abundant subtype of collagen found within dermal ECM connective tissue of human skin, followed by small amounts of type III collagen. Collagen precursor molecules (procollagen) are synthesized by dermal fibroblasts and are secreted into extracellular spaces, where it is enzymatically processed to mature collagen. Mature collagen spontaneously forms fibrils, which are stabilized by cross-links. Collagen fibrils are largely responsible for the strength and elasticity of skin. The half-life of collagen fibrils is about 15 years [41]. Therefore, fragmented collagen fibrils accumulate with the passage of time and have long-lasting consequences on skin structure and function. Breakdown of collagen is normally regulated by activity of MMPs and their natural inhibitors, tissue inhibitor of metalloproteinases (TIMPs). MMP-1 (collagenase) initiates cleavage of type I fibrillar and type III fibrillar at a single site within central triple helix. Once cleaved by MMP-1, collagen can be further degraded by MMP-3 (stromelysin) and MMP-9 (gelatinase). Elevated levels and activities of cutaneous MMPs are important in the development of age-related changes in skin [42].

3.2. Source of MMPs in human skin

In the skin, most of the epidermal cells are kerationocyte and dermal cells are fibroblast. In vitro data showed both keratinocyte and fibroblast can secrete MMPs, including MMP-1 (collagenase), MMP-3 (stromelysins) and MMP-9 (gelatinases). Cell culture and skin equivalent model studies have concluded that dermal fibroblasts are the major source of MMPs that are expressed in response to UV irradiation [43]. While, based on in situ hybridization and immunohistology, Fisher et al. reported that keratinocytes are the major cellular source of MMPs in UV-irradiated human skin in vivo [44]. They dissect epidermis and dermis from human skin by laser capture microdissection (LCM) and detect the MMP expression by real-time RT-PCR. MMP-1, 3 and 9 induced by 2 minimal erythema doses (MED) UV were primarily secreted by the epidermis, rather than dermis [41]. The reasons for the discrepancies between responses of human skin cells in vivo and responses of cultured skin cells in vitro are not well known. Although UV-induced MMPs (MMP-1, 3 and 9) are mainly produced by the epidermis, the secreted enzymes diffuse into the dermis and degrade collagen, as shown by in situ zymography [41]. Maybe dermal fibroblasts play a role in modulation of MMPs activities. It is also possible that dermal cells may also play a role in epidermal production of MMPs, through indirect paracrine mechanisms, by release of growth factors or cytokines, which in turn modulate MMP production by epidermal keratinocytes.

Besides keratinocytes and fibroblasts, neutrophil and macrophage are also important source of MMPs during UV irradiation or other pathological process in human skin. Fisher reported that MMP-8 (neutrophil collagenase) is present in human skin, 24 hours following UV irradiation, as a result of influx of neutrophils from the circulation [45]. Rijken et al. reported that neutrophils are major acute infiltrating cell in dermis after solar UV irradiation and these infiltrating neutrophils are a key source of in vivo MMP-1 and MMP-9 [46]. Keratinocytes and fibroblasts also produce MMPs but to a lesser extent [46]. Chung reported that macrophage-derived MMP-12 (macrophage elastase) mRNA maximally (11.9-fold) was induced by ultraviolet within 16 h in human skin in vivo [47]. Tewari confirmed that MMP-12 induction by UVA1 at 6 hours and contributing to elastin degeneration in late solar elastosis [48].

3.3. Role of MMPs in intrinsic skin ageing

Due to the limitation of experiment model for intrinsic ageing, details of molecular mechanism of MMP activation during chronological ageing are less clear than those in photoageing. Quan et al. screened basal mRNA expression levels of MMP family members in normal healthy, sun-protected, adult human skin. Among the 24 MMP genes in human beings, transcripts for MMP-8, 10, 12, 20 and 26 were not detected. Transcripts for other MMPs (MMP-1, 2, 3, 7, 9, 11, 13, 15, 16, 17, 19, 21, 22, 23, 24, 25, 27, 28) except MMP-14 were near the level of detection, approximately 1000-fold lower than internal control, housekeeping gene 36B4. Basal expression level of MMP-14 mRNA was approximately 35-fold higher than other detectable MMPs [41]. In both extrinsic and intrinsic ageing, elevated levels and activities of cutaneous MMPs have been demonstrated. MMP-1, MMP-2 and MMP-9 mRNA expressions are significantly elevated in sun-protected skin from patients older than 60 years of age compared with the 18- to 29-year-old age group [40, 49]. In parallel, aged skin was found to contain reduced levels of TIMPs both in normal skin and during acute wound repair [44]. Transcription factor AP-1 and $\alpha 2\beta 1$ integrin, which are key regulators of MMP-1 expression, are also elevated in fibroblasts in aged human skin in vivo [49]. In elder skin, reactive oxygen radicals produced during the mitochondrial oxidative energy metabolism, in particular in case of reduced antioxidant capacity, also contribute induction of MMPs [49, 50]. In addition, age-associated impaired ECM causes further fibroblast dysfunction in a self-sustaining loop. Fragmentation of collagen fibrils and collagen mass loss impairs fibroblast attachment with the collagenous ECM and then reduces spreading. The reduced mechanical force within fibroblast causes reduced collagen production from fibroblast and upregulates MMP expression especially MMP-1, which collectively causes further deterioration of the ECM [51–53]. In old cutaneous dermis, collagen fragmentation promotes oxidative stress and elevates MMP-1 production in fibroblasts from old skin [49]. Fibroblast cultured in three-dimensional collagen lattices with exogenous MMP-1 mimics the ECM microenvironment in old human dermis. And the fibroblast elevated levels of MMP-1, AP-1 and $\alpha 2\beta 1$ integrin and the antioxidant MitoQ can significantly reduce MMP-1 expression [49]. Reduced spreading/mechanical force of fibroblasts in aged skin induces MMP-1 expression through regulating c-Jun/AP-1 and elevating PGE2 production [53, 54]. The above studies reveal a novel mechanism by which alteration of fibroblast shape/mechanical force regulates MMP-1 expression through several pathways, such as c-JUN/AP-1, COX2-PGE and oxidative stress. Increasing mechanical force of old skin dermis by cross-linked hyaluronic acid filling can stimulate collagen synthesis and block MMP elevation partially [55].

3.4. Role of MMPs in photoageing

Both UVA and UVB can cause MMPs induction in human skin. In 1996, Fisher et al. first time showed induction of MMP mRNA expression and activities in human skin by low-dose UVB irradiation in vivo. Even 0.1 minimal erythema dose (MED) of UVB stimulates MMP expression and activities significantly. The 0.1 MED never causes perceptible erythema and is equivalent to 2–3 min solar irradiation on a summer day [56]. After UVB irradiation, the changes of AP-1 transcription factors became detectable within a few minutes and reached a maximum level at 60 min. Induction of MMP levels and activities was detectable approximately 16 hr.

post UVB irradiation, reached a maximum platform at 24 hr. and gradually disappeared after 48–72 h [56]. Usually, suberythemal dose of UV induces collagenase (MMP-1), a gelatinase (MMP-9) and a stromelysin (MMP-3) from keratinocytes and fibroblasts in vivo. High dose of UV irradiation induces more profound changes in MMPs expression and activity because it recruits more inflammatory cells, including neutrophil granulocytes, mast cells, monocytes-macrophages, lymphocytes and Langerhans cells [57, 58].

After UV irradiation, neutrophils are mainly MMP derived inflammatory cells and recruited in acute phase. Usually, neutrophil-derived MMPs are stored in granules ready for secretion [59]. Neutrophils can secrete MMP-1, MMP-8 and MMP-9. Macrophage-derived MMP-12 (macrophage elastase) mRNA maximally (11.9-fold) was induced by ultraviolet within 16 h in human skin in vivo [47]. Other UV-inducing MMPs like MMP-13, 10 and 7 are also reported.

The MMP induction was shown to be strongly dependent on the skin type: UVA or UVB/UVA irradiation of individuals with darkly pigmented skin resulted in only modest or little MMP induction, even if high UV dose was applied.

Among the UV-induced collagen, MMP-1 is the only enzyme able to initiate cleavage of collagen triple helix within type I and type III collagens, which are the two major fibril-forming molecules in the skin. Only the degrade fibrillar collagens initiate by MMP-1 can be cleaved by MMP-3 and MMP-9. The activity of MMP-1 remains under tight control even after UV irradiation [60]. After acute UV irradiation, only a small part of MMP-1 becomes active, whereas the majority of MMP-1 still inactive [60].

Besides MMP-1, MMP-8 (neutrophil collagenase) and MMP-13 (collagenase 3) also belong to collagenases being able to degrade native collagen without unwinding the triple helical assembly of the substrate [61]. They share similar configuration and enzymatic functions and only have small differences in substrate specificity. Recent studies suggest an induction of MMP-8 by UV irradiation but upregulation was minimal and plays a limited role in UV-mediated collagen damage in the skin [62]. MMP-13 shows less cleavage activity for type I collagen and type III collagen than MMP-1. However, it is 5–10 times more potent in cleaving type II collagen, a major collagen present in the cartilage [61]. Hence, MMP-8 and MMP-13 contribute very little to collagen damage in photoageing.

MMP-3 (stromelysin-1) and MMP-10 (stromelysin-2) belong to stromelysins, differ from collagenases and cannot digest intact type I collagen. They cleave various ECM proteins and are involved in the activation of pro-MMPs. The primary function of MMP-3 is the activation of pro-MMPs such as collagenases, gelatinase B and matrilysins during ECM turnover. In particular, the production of fully active MMP-3 is essential to partially activate pro-MMP-1 [61, 63, 64]. MMP-3 can degrade a large number of ECM proteins, such as type IV, V, IX and X collagens, gelatin, fibrillin-1, fibronectin, laminin and proteoglycans. The catalytic function of MMP-10 for type IV and type V collagens is quite weak compared to the MMP-3 activity [61, 65].

MMP-9 (gelatinase B or 92-kDa type IV collagenase) and MMP-2 (gelatinase A or 72-kDa type IV collagenase) belong to gelatinases, which can degrade type IV, V, VII and X collagens, fibronectin and elastin [64, 66]. They are essential in breakdown of fibrillar collagen fragments that initially cleaved by collagenases. In photoageing, MMP-9 mainly degrades type IV collagen, an important component of the cutaneous basement membrane [67].

Besides collagen impairment during photoageing, degrading of elastin also contributes to photoageing. Elastin constitutes only 2–4% of the total protein content of the skin; however, it is a major component that contributes to the function of recoil and resilience [68, 69]. UV-induced MMP-12 contributes to solar elastosis, which refers to the collection of dystrophic elastotic material in the dermis [48]. MMP-12 (macrophage metalloelastase) and MMP-7 (matrilysin) can degrade elastin efficiently after UV irradiation. MMP-12 is secreted by both macrophages and fibroblasts after UV irradiation. MMP-12 can cleave many other substrates belonging to the ECM, such as collagen type IV fragments, fibronectin, fibrillin-1, laminin, entactin, vitronectin, heparin and chondroitin sulphates. MMP-12 is also responsible for the activation of other pro-MMPs, such as pro-MMP1, MMP-2, MMP-3 and MMP-9 [61, 68]. MMP-7 can also cleave many other substrates of the ECM, such as collagen type IV, entactin, fibronectin, laminin and cartilage proteoglycan aggregates [61, 70].

Although UV is the most important factor causing extrinsic skin ageing, other factors such as smoking may also contribute to skin ageing through induction of MMPs. Indeed, it has been shown that tobacco smoking-induced MMP-1 causes extrinsic skin ageing in vivo [71].

MMPs induction by UV is related with reactive oxygen species (ROS). UV irradiation stimulates excess intracellular ROS including singlet oxygen, superoxide anion, hydrogen peroxide and hydroxyl radicals. ROS activates the mitogen-activated protein kinase (MAPK) family pathways. Then, transcription factors AP-1 and NF-κB are activated and regulated MMP-1, MMP-3 and MMP-9 resulting in the degradation of collagen [72, 73]. AP-1 also inhibits transforming growth factor-beta (TGF-β) signalling. TGF-β is an important regulator of type I procollagen synthesis in human skin [74]. Stimulation of MMP-1 and MMP-3 expression occurred via the upregulation of transcription factors AP-1 and NF-κB both in cultured keratinocytes and fibroblasts [75, 76]. AP-1 and MMP activities are also upregulated in the aged human skin in vivo [75]. Other influence factors generating ROS also induce AP-1- and NF-κB-mediated transcriptional activation and regulation of MMP gene expression. These pathways are shared by intrinsic and extrinsic skin ageing. Thus, even under physiological condition, low level of reactive oxygen species is constantly produced by the skin cells. The effects of ROS do not depend on their origin and all of them will lead to MMP activation and shift the MMP/TIMP balance. Treatment targeted to ROS generation can inhibit MMPs and prevent skin ageing. In recent years, it is demonstrated that many botanical supplements have effects of suppressing UV-B-induced ROS and MMPs expression, such as *Galla chinensis* [77], *Ixora parviflora* [78] and *Coffea Arabica* et al. [75].

There are a few medicines known to inhibit MMPs in human skin [51]. Topical application of tretinoin may suppress AP-1 and effectively inhibit a number of MMPs in both photoageing [44, 79] and intrinsic ageing [80]. Vitamin A antagonizes decreased cell growth and elevated collagen-degrading MMPs and stimulates collagen in aged skin. Doxycycline inhibits MMP activity at subantimicrobial doses used in many experimental systems. It is used clinically to treat periodontal disease. It is the only MMP inhibitor widely available clinically without major side effects [81]. Its topical application to the skin may also be beneficial against dermonecrosis induced by Loxosceles spider venom [82]. Interferon-γ and heparin have been reported inhibition of MMPs via inhibition of transcription levels.

3.5. Conclusion

MMPs are involved in various forms of skin ageing. It have been demonstrated that in both extrinsic and intrinsic ageing, reactive oxygen species are induced by physiological function of the organism or the extrinsic toxic effects like UV irradiation or tobacco smoking. Reactive oxygen species stimulate expression and activation of MMPs via AP-1 and NF-κB pathway. Meanwhile, MMP inhibitors and collagen synthesis are suppressed. MMPs can degrade all kinds of dermal ECM proteins such as collagen and elastin. Incomplete repair and chronic imbalance of ECM synthesis and degradation lead to disorganization of collagen and elastic fibres. The details of molecular events in skin ageing and MMP behaviours not completely understood. Although some MMP inhibitors are found to prevent skin ageing, more work should be done to reveal more mechanisms.

4. MMPs in skin cancer

Skin cancer is the most common type of malignancy, especially in the Caucasian population. There are three main types of skin cancers: basal cell carcinoma (BCC), squamous cell carcinoma (SCC) and cutaneous melanoma (CM). The first two together along with a number of less common skin cancers are known as non-melanoma skin cancer (NMSC) [83]. CM is the most aggressive, SCC is more likely to spread and BCC grows slowly and can also damage the tissue around. Two essential steps in tumour development are degradation of the basement membrane and invasion of the surroundings tissue by tumour cells, and MMPs maybe play an important role in them [84].

4.1. MMPs in cutaneous melanoma

CM is the most severe skin cancer characterized by a bad prognosis at metastatic stages due to resistance to most classical chemotherapies [85]. Degradation of basement membranes and ECM is an essential step in melanoma cell migration, invasion and metastasis formation. MMPs families are the main degrading substances involved in this process. Studies show that MMPs expression is not only restricted to tumour cells but also found in stromal cells. In addition to disrupt matrix proteins, MMPs can also cleave non-matrix components such as cytokines and growth factors. The modifications generated by the remodelling of matrix and non-matrix components can influence melanoma cell proliferation, adhesion, vascularization, survival, proteases expression and migration. The major findings about the expression and roles of some MMPs in melanoma are summarized according to their subgroup.

4.1.1. Collagenases

Three collagenases have been identified so far: collagenase 1 (MMP-1), collagenase 2 (MMP-8) and collagenase 3 (MMP-13) [84]. In 1980, MMP-1 was firstly detected in the stromal cells adjacent to melanoma metastases but not tumour cells and normal skin [86]. MMP-1 expression by stromal fibroblasts has also been implicated in the processing of PAR1, a thrombin receptor, thereby promoting the metastatic potential of cancer cells [87]. Their findings supported the hypothesis that collagenase facilitates connective tissue breakdown, which is associated with tumour invasiveness and metastatic spread. Further research found detection of MMP-1 at the edges of tumours and increased expression during melanoma progression [88]. Montgomery et al. found MMP-1 was also detected in a highly metastatic human melanoma cell line (M24met) together with MMP-2 and MMP-9 [89]. Furthermore, MMP-1 is detected in melanoma cells in advanced melanoma [90]. In terms of its expression, MMP-1 displays several promoter polymorphisms. Several studies had confirmed that the extra guanine (G) at -1607 bp was associated with enhanced transcription of MMP-1, increased enzymatic activity [91, 92] and also deep invasive melanoma [92]. Pearce et al. had assessed the functional effects of several single nucleotide polymorphisms (−1607GG > G, −839G > A, −755G > T, −519A > G, −422 T > A, −340C > T and 320C > T) on MMP1 gene promoter activity in cell lines of melanoma (A2058 and A375). Their results suggest that the polymorphisms exert haplotype effects on the transcriptional regulation of the MMP1 gene in cancer cells and indicate a need to examine haplotypes rather than any single polymorphism in genetic epidemiologic studies of the MMP1 gene in cancers [93]. The further research confirmed that the above polymorphisms correlate with ulceration patient status, but did not significantly associate with overall survival and other clinical factors [94], suggesting that MMP-1 promoter polymorphisms may individually or jointly play roles in the development of CM [95]. According to the literature, almost all the past studies showed that the expression of MMP-1 was positively correlated with melanoma invasion and metastases [96]. Nikkola et al. found the expression of collagenase-1 (MMP-1), stromelysin-1 (MMP-3) and collagenase-3 (MMP-13) in 70 melanoma metastases obtained from 56 patients treated with combined chemoimmunotherapy. They found that patients with MMP-1-positive metastases had significantly shorter disease-free survival compared to patients with MMP-1-negative metastases [97]. Despite a broad acceptance that MMP-1 plays a central role in invasion and metastasis, one study had found that high MMP-1 expression correlates with a favourable chemoimmunotherapy response in human metastatic melanoma [98].

In contrast to the other collagenases, MMP-8 had a very limited tissue distribution, thought to be restricted to neutrophils and chondrocytes. Giambernardi et al. firstly observed MMP-8 expression in human melanoma cells in 1998 [99]. This observation led them to assess in more detail the expression of MMP-8 in normal and malignant melanocytic cells. They found that MMP-8 was expressed by 11 of 12 human melanoma cell lines tested and all 10 primary melanomas examined, but was not expressed by four primary neonatal melanocyte strains. In contrast to its restricted tissue expression postpartum, MMP-8 was present in multiple embryonic tissues, including neural crest cells. The production of MMP-8 by migrating neural crest cells may contribute to their ability to degrade fibrillar collagen matrices while in transit [100]. Unlike the other MMPs, most studies showed that MMP-8 may have anti-tumour properties. Gutiérrez-Fernández et al. proposed that MMP-8 is a tumour protective factor, which also has the ability to reduce the metastatic potential of malignant cells in both mice and human [101]. In human melanoma, 23% somatic mutations of MMPs have been identified and 5 of these were found in the MMP-8 gene that lost thereby enzymatic activity [102]. MMP-8 gene variation might associate with an increased risk of malignant melanoma, which suggests that wild-type MMP-8 has the ability to inhibit melanoma progression, thus providing definitive evidence that MMP-8 is a tumour-suppressor gene [103]. On the controversy, high serum MMP-8 level is also associated with earlier recognized histopathology markers of melanoma progression and haematogenous spreading of melanoma through vascular invasion [104]. Although Syrjänen et al. had reported that patients with high serum MMP-8 levels may benefit from adjuvant IFN-α therapy [105], Prošvicová et al. reported that MMP-8 does not seem to function as a tumour suppressor in the most recent study [106]. In all, MMP-8 seems to have two different effects and needs further investigation in the future.

MMP-13 was shown to be expressed during invasive vertical growth phase of melanoma, but its expression is higher when the tumour starts to invade surrounding tissues [88]. Further studies also confirmed MMP-13 involved in BCC progression, invasion and metastasis [107, 108]. Moreover, MMP-13 can also mediate melanocytes and melanoma growth in vitro studies [109]. To confirm the role of stroma-derived MMP-13 in the invasion process, Zigrino et al. also investigated the invasiveness of melanoma cells upon intradermal injection in mice with complete inactivation of MMP-13. Their data suggest an important role of MMP-13 in tumour growth and an unexpected role in organ-specific metastasis of melanoma cells [110]. The recent research showed that MMP-13 has a dual effect in melanoma, as it promotes invasion and metastasis by cleaving laminin-5 (Ln-5) into small fragments but disrupts vasculogenic mimicry formation [111]. However, host-derived MMP-13 exhibits a protective role in lung metastasis of melanoma cells by local endostatin production [112].

4.1.2. Gelatinases

MMP-2 and MMP-9, also known as gelatinases A and B, were detected by immunohistochemical staining in stromal and/or melanocytic cells in melanoma [113] and stromal cells as the major source for it [114]. Using in situ enzymatic assays, proteolytic activity of MMP-2 and MMP-9 was predominantly localized in peritumoural areas while no activity was observed within the tumour cell nests [115]. MMP-2 cleaves fibronectin into small fragments to enhance the adhesion and migration of human melanoma cells [116]. There is growing evidence that MMP-2 is an important factor for promoting cancer cell invasion and independent predictive factor for lymph node involvement [117]. The pro-tumour function of several molecules (NADPH oxidase 1 [118], angiotensin II [119], hyaluronan-binding protein 1 [120], osteopontin [121] and interleukin-8 [122]) was also MMP2-dependent. The expression of MMP-2 in CM could be a useful diagnostic and prognostic indicator in melanoma [123, 124]. However, MMP-2 serum level appears to be of limited clinical value in monitoring [125, 126]. At the genetic level, functional promoter polymorphisms −1306 C/T and −735 C/T were known to modify the gene transcription but not associated with melanoma progression [127].

Among all the members of the MMP family, MMP-9 is of crucial importance in tumour invasion and metastasis. MMP-9 was significantly higher in melanoma patients than in controls [128]. Transfection of sense MMP-9 can enhance growth and invasion of melanoma cells, further confirming its important role in tumour invasion and metastasis [129]. MMP-9 may also act as tumour suppressor by processing matrix macromolecules. Enzymatic activity of MMP-9 towards the basement membrane collagen type IV was shown to generate a proteolytic active fragment, tumstatin, which suppresses activity of endothelial cells and inhibits pathological angiogenesis [130]. Circulating MMP-9 levels had shown low sensitivity and specificity and did not seem to be good tumour markers in patients with melanoma [131].

Nikkola et al. reported that MMP-1, MMP-9 and MMP-13 play important roles at different phases of metastatic melanoma spread and serum MMP-9 could particularly have clinical value in identifying patients at high risk for melanoma progression [132]. There was no strong evidence that MMP-9 SNPs play a role in melanoma progression [133].

4.1.3. Stromelysins

MMP-3, MMP-10 and MMP-11 correspond to stromelysins 1, 2 and 3, respectively. MMP-3, also called stromelysin-1, was one of the first proteinases found to be associated with cancer. MMP-3 was localized to the deeper margins of human melanoma [134] and confirmed to correlate with shorter disease-free survival [97]. However, Tas et al. proposed that neither of the serum levels of MMP-3 could be a good indicator of invasion and metastasis nor can be recommended as a tumour marker in the management of melanoma patients owing to lack of sensitivity and specificity by detecting serum MMP-3 levels in 70 patients with cutaneous malignant melanoma [135]. At the genetic level, functional promoter polymorphisms −1171 5A/6A was known to modify the gene transcription [127], but no strong evidence provided into the role of the MMP3 variants in melanoma progression [127, 136]. More researches are needed to confirm it specific roles in CM. Studies on the other two stromelysins, MMP-10 and MMP-11, in CM were very limited. It seems that the stromelysins are involved in the generalized growth and expansion of the neoplastic cell mass [107], but the possible correlation with CM is still unclear. MMP-11 is a fibroblastic factor expressed in stromal cells adjacent to carcinoma cells, but was not found in human melanoma [137].

4.1.4. Matrilysins

MMP-7 and MMP-26 belong to the group of matrilysins. Matrilysin (MMP-7) is expressed in various types of malignant tumours. Kawasaki et al. found MMP-7 expression in primary melanomas and in metastatic melanomas, but not in common naevi or Spitz naevi. Their observations indicate that MMP-7 may be associated with melanoma progression and may enhance melanoma tumour cell invasion [138]. However, a direct role for MMP-7 in melanoma development has not been shown. MMP-26 was not generally expressed in melanoma cells [139] but elevated in melanoma tissues, and it may serve as a molecular marker for the early diagnosis of melanoma [140].

4.1.5. MT-MMPs

Two types of MT-MMPs exist: four type I transmembrane proteins (MMP-14, MMP-15, MMP-16 and MMP-24) and two glycosylphosphatidylinositol (GPI)-anchored proteins (MMP-17 and MMP-25). MT1-MMP, also referred to as MMP-14, was the first discovered membrane-type MMP [141]. MT1-MMP expressing clones can induce rapid tumour growth and high tumour vascularization in nude mice [142]. It is expressed in tumour cells mainly at the leading edge of the invasive front of melanomas [115] and can serve as prognostic factor as its expression strongly associates with cancer progression and metastasis and poor prognosis of patients [143]. Activation of MMP-2 is mediated by binding to the complex of MT1-MMP with tissue inhibitor of MMP-2 (TIMP-2) on the cell surface [144]. Further study suggested that activation of MMP2 by MT1-MMP is required to sustain RAC1 activity and promote MT1-MMP-dependent cell motility. These data highlight a novel MT1-MMP/MMP2/RAC1 signalling axis in melanoma that may represent an intriguing molecular target for the treatment of invasive melanoma [145]. Moreover, MT1-MMP can activate Notch1 in melanoma cells by directly cleave it to induce melanoma growth [146]. Recently, MT1-MMP has been found to also modulate gene expression. Shaverdashvili et al. identified the tumour suppressor gene SPRY4 as a new transcriptional target of MT1-MMP and a novel molecular effector of MT1-MMP that affect melanoma cell motility [147]. MMP-2 is considered to be activated by MT-MMPs and its expression in melanoma cells was involved in the degradation of ECM during melanoma growth and correlated with later melanoma metastasis. Thus, MT-MMPs and MMP-2 cooperate in the invasive and metastatic process of melanoma cells [123]. Recent research also showed that effective inhibition of MT1-MMP and MMP2 can effectively reduce melanoma cell growth, migration and invasion in vitro [148]. The information could help in developing new therapies designed to interfere with MMPs activation and management of cancer and metastases.

The expression of MT2-MMP (MMP-15) and MT3-MMP (MMP-16) was generally increased in primary and metastatic melanoma cells. A consistent colocalization of MT2-MMP/MMP-2 and MT3-MMP/MMP-2 in the nodular melanoma and metastatic melanoma cells was found by double immunofluorescence [123]. MT3-MMP was significantly upregulated in biopsies of human melanoma metastases and induced efficient invasion of the cells in fibrin, a provisional matrix component frequently found at tumour-host tissue interfaces and perivascular spaces of melanoma, which suggest that MT3-MMP functions as a matrix composition-dependent effector of melanoma cell invasion [149]. Further study showed that overexpression of MT3-MMP in human melanoma is associated with poor clinical outcome, collagen bundle assembly around tumour cell nests and lymphatic invasion [150]. So far, there is no report of MMP-17 and MMP-25 related to melanoma. Although more studies are required to unveil the roles of GPI-MT-MMPs in cancer, the data so far obtained suggest that these proteases influence cancer progression by mechanisms that are different from the TM-MT-MMPs. First, GPI-MTMMPs do not act as progelatinase activators; second, their ECM degradation profile appears to be very limited; third, GPI-MT-MMPs do not promote tumour cell migration and invasion and fourth, their inhibition profile appears unique [61].

4.1.6. Other MMPs

MMP-12, MMP-19, MMP-20, MMP-21, MMP-23, MMP-27 and MMP-28 have not been catalogued in any of the subgroups mentioned above. Zhang et al. found that MMP-12 expression in melanoma was significantly associated with tumour invasion and metastasis [151]. Müller et al. found that MMP19 expression was upregulated in the vertical growth phase and in metastases (mainly expressed close to tumour surrounding fibroblasts), suggesting participation of MMP19 in melanoma development and MMP19 as a candidate marker for identifying vertical growth phase melanoma and metastatic melanomas [152]. MMP-21 is upregulated at early stages of melanoma progression but disappears with more aggressive phenotype, suggesting expression of MMP-21 may serve as a marker of malignant transformation of melanocytes and does not associate with the presence of micrometastases [139]. Moogk et al. confirmed that MMP-23 was expressed in human melanoma by detecting MMP-23 expression in primary melanoma patients who received adjuvant immunotherapy. The results showed an inverse association between primary melanoma MMP-23 expression and the anti-tumour T cell response, suggesting MMP-23 is a potential immunosuppressive target in melanoma [153]. MMP-28 was not generally expressed in melanoma cells [139]. To date, there was no report relating to MMP-27 and melanoma.

4.2. MMPs in basal cell carcinoma

BCC is the most common cancer in white-skinned individuals with increasing incidence rates worldwide. There are different histopathological subtypes, of which nodular is the most frequent, followed by superficial and infiltrative, and mixed types are frequently found as well. Most BCC occur in the head and neck region (i.e. sun-exposed), followed by trunk and extremities (i.e. relatively sun-unexposed) [154]. Although BCC is characterized by slow progression and low metastatic potential, it has a propensity to be locally destructive. If untreated, BCC may invade subcutaneous fat, muscles and even bones [154]. The invasion of tumour cells is a complex, multistage process, which is governed by complex interactions between various biomarkers, especially MMPs, cell-cell adhesion molecules (such as β-catenin) and chemokine receptor-ligand complexes (SDF-1/CXCR4) [155, 156].

4.2.1. Collagenases

MMP-1 is the primary collagenolytic enzyme in BCC and expressed at various intensities in epithelial tumour cells and surrounding stromal cells, including fibroblasts, inflammatory cells and vascular endothelial cells [157, 158]. The expression of MMP-1 is significantly enhanced at the invasive front of BCC, suggesting its role in the initial steps of tumour proliferation; even when potentially important variables such as age and individual variability are controlled for, tumour-specific effects on the expression of MMP-9 and MMP-1 also need be taken into consideration [159]. In order to determine correlations between invasiveness and histologic differentiation, the expression of MMP-1, MMP-3, Ki-67, p53, EGFR and CD44v6 was detected in 108 cases of BCC using tissue array. The results showed that the loss of palisading arrangement in BCC was correlated with the MMP-1 expression of stromal cells [160]. Odds ratio for development of morpheaform and recurrent BCC was 6.2 for positive MMP-1 immunostaining in epithelial tumour cells, suggesting MMP-1 is associated with morpheaform and recurrent BCC [161]. MMP-13 is involved in the degradation of ECM and its expression is associated with malignant transformation in skin carcinogenesis [155, 162]. The expression of MMP-13 is not confined to tumour cells alone, as its expression is also upregulated in stromal cells surrounding epithelial tumours, including fibroblasts, inflammatory cells and endothelial cells [163]. The further study found endothelial cells-derived MMP-13 is associated with endothelial cell proliferation and vascular differentiation, suggesting MMP-13 maybe is an efficient therapeutic target for future treatment of BBC [162]. The CXCR4 ligand, stromal cell-derived factor 1 alpha (SDF-1α), directed BCC invasion and that this was mediated by gelatinase activity of MMP-13 [155]. By immunohistochemistry, MMP-13 was detected in the cytoplasm of the malignant cells and occasionally in the surrounding stromal cells. Statistical analysis showed no significant association between MMP-13 immunostaining and patients or tumour characteristics, but the expression of MMP-13 was more intense in the epithelial tumour cells located at the invading front [164]. Taken together, MMP-13 expression may serve as a prognostic marker for early tumour invasiveness and also an increased risk for BCC recurrence. Neutrophils are a major source of MMP-8. MMP-8 was indeed detected in BCC, but its source is more problematic as it diffusely presented only throughout the stroma. It is reasonable to suggest that circulating neutrophils present in the tissue at the time of biopsy might be responsible for this enzyme, but this does not rule out contributions by resident neutrophils [157].

4.2.2. Gelatinases

MMP-2 and MMP-9 play an important role in the development, progression, invasion and metastasis of BCC and proposed to be used as prognostic factors of BCC [165]. MMP-2 is a leading ECM degrading protease and upregulates in almost all cancers by creating a suitable microenvironment for the proliferation of cancer cells and epithelial-mesenchymal transition (EMT) [61]. MMP-2 is mostly secreted by stromal cells surrounding BCC tumours and rarely by keratinocytes and BCC tumour cells [166]. MMP-2 expression may contribute to the distinct invasive patterns seen in BCC as its expression was higher in the stroma of high-risk BCC when compared to low-risk BCC [167]. MMP-9 has been historically identified as a basement membrane degrading protease, due to its high affinity for collagen IV. Experimental models, mostly based on MMP-9 knockout mice, have provided unequivocable evidences about the pivotal role played by the enzyme in tumour growth, invasiveness and angiogenesis [61]. MMP-9 prominently expressed at the invading edge of the BCC and was mostly secreted by inflammatory cells, such as macrophages, rather than by tumour cells [158, 168]. Odds ratio for development of morpheaform and recurrent BCC was 5.8 for positive MMP-9 immunostaining in tumour stroma, suggesting MMP-9 expression in stromal cells is associated with morpheaform and recurrent BCC [161]. In order to compare the expressions of mRNA for metalloproteinases (MMP-2 and MMP-9) and type IV collagen in BCC and normal tissues from the tumour interface, Goździalska et al. detected the expressions of mRNA for MMP-2, MMP-9 and type IV collagen by RT-PCR. They revealed that MMP-2 and MMP-9 expressed significantly higher in nodular and infiltrative BCC than normal tissues adjacent to tumours, suggesting that MMP-2 and MMP-9 could be used as prognostic factors of BCC [165].

4.2.3. Stromelysins

MMP-10 was entirely negative in premalignant lesions and only detected in epithelial cancer cells. By statistical analysis, MMP-10 expression does not correlate with the invasive behaviour of tumours as assessed by their histology, but may be induced by the wound healing and inflammatory matrix remodelling events associated with skin tumours [169, 170]. MMP-11 seems to be associated with benign fibroblastic tumours and is a fibroblastic factor expressed in stromal cells adjacent to carcinoma cells. Thewes et al. found MMP-11 only expressed in fibroblasts surrounding malignant epithelial tumour cells in more than half of BCC. Of interest, different percentages of positive immunoreactivity were found between the lowest level

(29.4%) in the nodular-ulcerative subgroup and the highest level (65.4%) in the morpheaform subgroup [171].

4.2.4. *Matrilysins*

Expression of MMP-7 is low in the normal epidermis and is induced by physiological processes such as wound healing, but also malignant transformation of epidermal cells. Hartmann-Petersen et al. revealed that the intensity of MMP-7 was found in tumour cells of BCC. Furthermore, the activity of MMP-7 was associated with the hyaluronan (HA) receptor CD44 and its staining intensity was inversely correlated with that of CD44 in BCC [172]. MMP-26 expression is barely detected in BCC epithelium or stromal cells and is therefore not considered significant in the development of BCC nor in the process of angiogenesis [168, 173].

4.2.5. *MT-MMPs*

MT-MMP acts as a membrane activator of other soluble MMPs, such as MMP-2 [156, 167]. Oh et al. has detected MT1-MMP expression in various histological subtypes of BCC. The results showed that MT1-MMP immunoreactivity was increased in the high-risk BCC and at the invading front of mixed BCC tumour islands, suggesting MT1-MMP might be a novel marker for high-risk BCC [156].

4.2.6. *Other MMPs*

In BCC, MMP-12 was more often found in macrophages than in cancer cells, indicating that the level of human MMP-12 expression correlates with epithelial dedifferentiation and histologic aggressiveness [174]. MMP-21 protein was not detected in normal adult skin. However, it was present in invasive cancer cells of aggressive subtypes of basal and SCC [175].

4.3. MMPs in cutaneous squamous cell carcinoma

SCC is the second most common type of NMSC and characterized by malignant proliferation of epidermal keratinocytes. Its incidence rates appear to be increasing in many populations of European heritage [176]. Evidently, the primary cause of cutaneous SCC is cumulative lifetime sun exposure (especially UVB). Furthermore, ionizing radiation, immune suppression, chronic inflammation and human papillomavirus (HPV) infection may lead to the development of SCC. The prognostic risk factors include diameter, depth of invasion, histologic differentiation, rapid growth, anatomic site, immune suppression and etiology, so that tumours arising from scars and chronic ulcers tend to be aggressive [176]. Unlike BCC, SCC exhibits an increased risk of metastasis, although the rate of metastasis is much lower than that of melanoma [177]. Like BCC, MMPs also play an important role in the degradation of ECM and basement membrane [84].

4.3.1. *Collagenases*

MMP-1 mRNA was detected in tumour cells and/or in stromal cells in all cases of SCC, its expression could be an early event in the development of SCC [178]. Ultraviolet radiation may cause NMSC. In order to find out if UV irradiation modulates the expression of MMPs, Ramos et al. investigated it and found MMP-1 was upregulated 4 h after UVA and 16 h after UVB irradiation of tumour cells [179]. Further clinical research revealed that MMP-1 is a significant marker associated with the invasiveness of SCC and also a poor clinical outcome. Thus, it will be helpful to evaluate the invasiveness by measuring the expression of MMP-1 in SCC [160]. Specific expression of MMP-13 by SCC cells in vitro and in vivo strongly suggests a role for MMP-13 in the high invasion capacity of SCC cells [180]. In patients with recessive dystrophic epidermolysis bullosa, MMP-13 expression is strongly positive in SCC but negative in benign hyperkeratotic lesions, suggesting MMP13 may be a useful differentiating marker between SCC and benign hyperkeratotic lesions [181]. Further studies showed that MMP-13 is also involved in the maintenance of angiogenesis through the release of VEGF from the tumour ECM [182]. Taken together, MMP-1 and MMP-13 are expressed mainly in stromal cells, particularly in tumour-associated fibroblast. Both MMP-1 and MMP-13 can cleave native fibrillar collagen and remodel the ECM thereby play a crucial role in tumour progression in vivo [183]. MMP-8 expressed in tissue from head and neck carcinomas, but the amount of MMP-8 in them is rather low [184]. Further study found that MMP-8 was positive in peritumoural inflammatory cells in cutaneous SCC, but it was not associated with the overall survival of patients with cutaneous SCC [185].

4.3.2. Gelatinases

The expression of MMP-2 greatly increased in tumour stroma and parenchyma of SCC and may contribute to the distinct invasive patterns seen in SCC [167]. MMP-9 showed positive staining mainly in the granular layer of normal epidermis. While in SCC and BD, MMP-9 showed positive staining in the dysplastic lesions even in the basal layer [186]. Borchers et al. reported that interactions between malignant keratinocytes and adjacent stromal fibroblasts are critical in directing expression of MMP-9 to the tumour-stroma interface in human SCC tumours [187], and also MMP-9 was found to be focally expressed by neoplastic epithelial cells of cutaneous carcinomas at the infiltrative edges in microinvasive carcinomas and in dyskeratotic foci in Bowen's disease and widely invasive carcinomas [188]. The expression of MMP9 was higher in SCC compared to BCC and AK [189], and also may contribute to the more aggressive behaviour of SCC in immunosuppressed patients [190]. Nan et al. observed that the MMP9 Arg668Gln polymorphism was significantly associated with a decreased risk of SCC, but no correlation to BCC and melanoma [191]. The reduced expression of collagen IV combined with an increased expression of both MMP2 and MMP9 could account for the increased metastatic potential of SCC vs. BCC through an increased invasion of the ECM and the vascular space [192]. To investigate the expression of MMP-2 and MMP-9 in NMSC and compare their expression between different tumour types with clinicopathological factors, a study of 11 normal skin, 29 Bowen's disease and 40 SCC samples for MMP-2 and MMP-9 expression was carried out using immunohistochemistry and in situ hybridization. The results showed that there was a correlation between increased metalloproteinase expression and depth of lesion (MMP-2), inflammation (MMP-2 and MMP-9) and microvessel density (MMP-2 and MMP-9) [193]. These results provided additional evidence of the role of MMP-2 and MMP-9 in tumour invasiveness of keratinocyte-derived tumours.

4.3.3. Stromelysins

MMP-3 or stromelysin-1 is induced in the tumour stroma in the early stages of tumourigenesis. It can degrade a variety of matrix and non-matrix molecules such as growth factors,

HB-EGF and E-cadherin. Fibroblast-derived MMP-3 is a necessary mediator of tumour vascularization and tumour progression and thus plays an important role in mechanisms that modulate tumour metastasis [194]. The expression of MMP-3 was increased in both tumour cells and stromal cells in metastatic SCC and also correlated to that of MMP-1 localized at tumour mass and stroma of the invasive SCC [178]. McCawley et al. demonstrated that MMP3-null animals have an increased sensitivity to the development of SCC, suggesting that MMP3 has a protective role in SCC. However, not all cellular responses affected by a loss of MMP3 are tumour-protective, and tumour expression of MMP3 is coincident with an invasive tumour phenotype. Transgenic mice were generated with MMP3 targeted to keratinocytes to examine the biological role of tumour-produced MMP3 in their further study. Overexpression of MMP3 reduced tumour multiplicity in response to chemically induced SCC. Vascular density was increased with MMP3 overexpression; however, other cellular processes, including tumour growth and leukocyte infiltration, were unaffected. These studies suggest that keratinocyte expression of MMP3 promotes cellular differentiation, impeding tumour establishment during tumourigenesis [194]. MMP-10 or stromelysin-2, similar to other metalloproteases, facilitates the recruitment of infiltrating cells by remodelling the ECM. Moreover, MMP-10 upregulates several other MMPs such as MMP-1, MMP-7, MMP-9 and MMP-13 that are essential for tumour progression. The function of this protease is restricted to the initial process of tumour initiation, indicating that it might not be important in invasion or metastasis [13]. In 2001, MMP-10 was only detected in epithelial laminin-5 positive cancer cells in SCC, and its expression does not correlate with the invasive behaviour of tumours [169]. More precisely, MMP-10 is highly expressed in SCC stromal cells and is upregulated by tumour-associated cytokines, including TGF-β and TNF-α. The level of MMP-10 expression in tumour epithelium of grades III and II of SCC was significantly greater compared to grade I tumours [195]. Recently, Kadeh et al. also found high immunohistochemical expression of MMP-10 in tumour epithelium and stroma in SCC. Moreover, they also confirmed that the level of MMP-10 expression in tumour epithelium of grades III and II of SCC was significantly greater compared to grade I tumours [170]. Thus, MMP-10 was highly expressed in both tumour epithelium and stromal cells and may play a role in the initial stages of SCC progression [13], but does not correlate with the invasive behaviour of SCC [169]. MMP-11 found a positive immunoreactivity in fibroblasts surrounding malignant epithelial tumour cells in 4 of 25 (16%) SCCs, whereas the tumour cells themselves were negative [171]. Besides the above report, there was no other MMP-11-related study in SCC was found. Thus, the role of MMP-11 involved in SCC maybe so limited.

4.3.4. Matrilysins

MMP-7 can digest a wide range of ECM proteins and cleave several cell surface proteins, including E-cadherin and syndecan-1 [196]. In addition to enhance tumour invasion and metastasis directly, MMP-7 also exerts indirect effects through the activation of MMP-2 and MMP-9 [197]. Mitsui et al. found that the expression of MMP7 increased in invasive SCC and its expression was induced by IL-24. Moreover, blocking of MMP7 by a specific antibody significantly delayed the migration of SCC cells in culture. These results suggest that MMP-7 in SCC is derived by IL-24 and may play a role in SCC invasion [198]. MMP-7 was present in tumour cells and mainly located in the invasive front, suggesting play a role in promoting the growth of cutaneous SCC [199]. MMP-26 is predominantly located in pre- and early-invasive areas in SCC and plays an essential role in the initial stages of skin cancer [200]. In addition, MMP-26 can also stimulate MMP-9 expression [190]. MMP-26 is upregulated in keratinocytes during early skin carcinogenesis and becomes downregulated during histological dedifferentiation of SCC. Thus, lack of MMP-26 in SCC could be a marker of aggressive growth [37].

4.3.5. MT-MMPs

MT1-MMP or MMP-14 plays an important role in the degradation of various ECM proteins and in activating pro-MMP-2 [201]. MMP-14 mRNA was detected both in epithelial cancer cells and stromal fibroblasts [169]. MMP-14 showed a statistically significant linear trend with decreasing values for tumoural and stromal expression with invasion suggesting that it might be of use as a prognosticator [202]. Both stromal fibroblasts and tumour cells in SCC, particularly at the invasive front of the tumour, secrete MMP-14. MMP-14 in tumour cells can induce tumour cell invasion, whereas MMP-14 in fibroblasts may be important in the stromal response to tumour cells that characterize the desmoplastic reaction [203].

4.3.6. Other MMPs

Several other MMPs are reported to be involved in the pathophysiology of SCC. MMP-12 expression by tumour cells in SCC of the vulva correlates with invasiveness, while macrophage-derived MMP-12 in tumour predicts better outcome. These results suggest a dual role for MMP-12 in tumour progression [204]. Unlike most MMPs, MMP-19 was present in the hyperproliferative (p63-positive), E-cadherin-negative epidermis at the tumour surface but downregulated in invasive cancer islands in SCC, suggesting MMP-19 maybe a protective factor and preventing the occurrence of SCC [205]. MMP-21, the newest member of the MMP gene family, has been suggested to play an important role in embryogenesis and tumour progression and to be a target of the Wnt, Pax and Notch signalling pathways. MMP-21 is present in invasive cancer cells of SCC and is upregulated by TGF-beta1 in keratinocytes [175]. It may be involved in keratinocyte differentiation but does not associate with invasion of SCC [13]. MMP-28 is the newest member of the matrix metalloproteinase enzyme family. Unlike many other MMPs, MMP-28 was not detected in the invading cancer cell nests of squamous cell cancers of various grades.

4.4. Conclusion

MMPs play an important role in tumour development, growth, angiogenesis and metastasis. Each of these proteinases has specific roles in determining the invasive capacity of the tumour. The expression and role of various MMPs in BCC, BCC and SCC were summarized in **Tables 1–3**. Different MMPs might form a network, in which each has a distinct role in the cleavage of a particular matrix component or activation of other MMPs. Stromal cells are the major source of MMPs, but tumour cells, fibroblasts and inflammatory cells all express a distinct set of MMPs capable of complementing the proteolysis needed in tumour progression. Hence, the function of distinct MMPs and their regulation should be considered the principal targets for development of antineoplastic drugs or chemotherapeutic agents.

Member	Expression	Role
Collagenases		
MMP-1	Expressed by stromal fibroblasts adjacent to melanoma metastases and also melanoma cells in advanced melanoma	Promotes progression, invasion and metastatic
MMP-8	Expressed by melanoma cells	Two different effects: (1) Tissue expressed MMP-8 inhibits melanoma progression; (2) Serum MMP-8 is a marker of melanoma progression and haematogenous spreading of melanoma through vascular invasion
MMP-13	Expressed by melanoma cells	A dual effect: (1) Stroma-derived MMP-13 promotes progression, invasion and metastatic; (2) Host-derived MMP-13 exhibits a protective role in lung metastasis
Gelatinases		
MMP-2	Expressed by stromal and/or melanocytic cells in melanoma, and stromal cells as the major source	Promotes cancer cell invasion and independent predictive factor for lymph node involvement
MMP-9	Expressed by stromal and/or melanocytic cells in melanoma, and stromal cells as the major source	Promotes invasion and metastatic
Stromelysins		
MMP-3	Expressed in deeper margins of human melanoma	Correlates with shorter disease-free survival
MMP-10	Expressed by malignant melanomas, especially in the ECM adjacent to blood vessels	Role was very limited
MMP-11	Expressed in stromal cells adjacent to carcinoma cells	Role was very limited
Matrilysins		
MMP-7	Expressed in primary melanomas and in metastatic melanomas	Promotes progression and invasion
MMP-26	Elevated in melanoma tissues, but not in melanoma cells	May serve as a molecular marker for the early diagnosis of melanoma
MT-MMPs		
MMP-14	Expressed by tumour cells mainly at the leading edge of the invasive front of melanomas	Strongly associates with cancer progression and metastasis and poor prognosis of patients
MMP-15	Expressed in primary and metastatic melanoma cells	Promotes invasion and associates with poor clinical outcome
MMP-16	Expressed in primary and metastatic melanoma cells	Promotes invasion and associates with poor clinical outcome
MMP-17	None reported to date	Unknown
MMP-24	None reported to date	Unknown
MMP-25	None reported to date	Unknown

Member	Expression	Role
Other MMPs		
MMP-12	Mainly expressed by tumour cells	Promotes invasion and metastatic
MMP-19	Upregulated in the vertical growth phase and in metastases (mainly expressed close to tumour surrounding fibroblasts)	Serves as a candidate marker for identifying vertical growth phase melanoma and metastatic melanomas
MMP-20	None reported to date	Unknown
MMP-21	Upregulated at early stages of melanoma progression but disappears with more aggressive phenotype	Serves as a marker of malignant transformation of melanocytes
MMP-23	Expressed by melanoma cells and also fibroblasts surrounding melanoma islands	Inversely associates with the anti-tumour T cell response
MMP-27	None reported to date	Unknown
MMP-28	Not generally expressed in melanoma cells	Unknown

Table 1. The expression and roles of MMPs in cutaneous melanoma.

Member	Expression	Role
Collagenases		
MMP-1	Expressed at various intensities in epithelial tumour cells and surrounding stromal cells including fibroblasts, inflammatory cells and vascular endothelial cells	Plays a role in the initial steps of tumour proliferation and associates with morpheaform and recurrent BCC
MMP-8	Diffusely presented throughout the stroma	Unknown
MMP-13	Expressed by epithelial tumour cells and stromal cells including fibroblasts, inflammatory cells and vascular endothelial cells	Serves as a prognostic marker for early tumour invasiveness and an increased risk for BCC recurrence
Gelatinases		
MMP-2	Mostly secreted by stromal cells surrounding BCC tumours	Plays an important role in the development, progression, invasion and metastasis
MMP-9	Expressed at the invading edge of the BCC and was mostly secreted by inflammatory cells such as macrophages, rather than by tumour cells	Plays an important role in the development, progression, invasion and metastasis
Stromelysins		
MMP-3	None reported to date	Unknown
MMP-10	Expressed by epithelial cancer cells	Maybe induced by the wound healing and inflammatory matrix remodelling events associated with skin tumours
MMP-11	Expressed by fibroblasts surrounding malignant epithelial tumour cells	Unknown

Member	Expression	Role
Matrilysins		
MMP-7	Expressed by tumour cells	Maybe associated with poor differentiation
MMP-26	Not expressed in BCC	Unknown
MT-MMPs		
MMP-14	Expressed by tumour cells mainly at the invading front of mixed BCC tumour islands	Serves as a novel marker for high-risk BCC
MMP-15	None reported to date	Unknown
MMP-16	None reported to date	Unknown
MMP-17	None reported to date	Unknown
MMP-24	None reported to date	Unknown
MMP-25	None reported to date	Unknown
Other MMPs		
MMP-12	More often found in macrophages than in cancer cells	Correlates with epithelial dedifferentiation and histologic aggressiveness
MMP-19	None reported to date	Unknown
MMP-20	None reported to date	Unknown
MMP-21	Presents in invasive cancer cells of aggressive subtypes	Maybe promote invasion
MMP-23	None reported to date	Unknown
MMP-27	None reported to date	Unknown
MMP-28	None reported to date	Unknown

Table 2. The expression and roles of MMPs in BCC.

Member	Expression	Role
Collagenases		
MMP-1	Expressed by tumour cells and stromal cells, mainly in stromal cells	Served as a significant marker associated with the invasiveness of SCC and also a poor clinical outcome
MMP-8	Lowly expressed by peritumoural inflammatory cells in SCC	Role is limited
MMP-13	Expressed by tumour cells and/or stromal cells, mainly in stromal cells	Promotes invasion and angiogenesis
Gelatinases		
MMP-2	Expressed by tumour stroma and parenchyma	Promotes invasion
MMP-9	Expressed in the tumour-stroma interface of SCC and also at the infiltrative edges of microinvasive carcinomas	Promotes invasion and metastatic

Member	Expression	Role
Stromelysins		
MMP-3	Expressed by tumour stroma at the early stages of tumourigenesis and upregulated in both tumour cells and stromal cells in metastatic SCC	Promotes progression, invasion and metastatic
MMP-10	Highly expressed in stromal cells	Promotes progression
MMP-11	Expressed by fibroblasts surrounding tumour cells	Role is limited
Matrilysins		
MMP-7	Expressed by tumour cells and mainly located in the invasive front	Promotes invasion and metastatic
MMP-26	Upregulated in keratinocytes during early skin carcinogenesis and becomes downregulated during histological dedifferentiation of SCC	Plays an essential role in the initial stages of SCC
MT-MMPs		
MMP-14	Detected both in epithelial cancer cells and stromal fibroblasts	Promotes invasion
MMP-15	None reported to date	Unknown
MMP-16	None reported to date	Unknown
MMP-17	None reported to date	Unknown
MMP-24	None reported to date	Unknown
MMP-25	None reported to date	Unknown
Other MMPs		
MMP-12	Expressed by tumour cells and macrophages	A dual role: Expressed by tumour cells correlates with invasiveness, while macrophage-derived MMP-12 in tumour predicts better outcome
MMP-19	Expressed by the hyperproliferative, E-cadherin-negative epidermis at the tumour surface but downregulated in invasive cancer islands	Maybe a protective factor and prevent the occurrence of SCC
MMP-20	None reported to date	Unknown
MMP-21	Expressed by invasive cancer cells of SCC	Promotes progression and invasion
MMP-23	None reported to date	Unknown
MMP-27	None reported to date	Unknown
MMP-28	None expression in SCC	Unknown

Table 3. The expression and roles of MMPs in cutaneous SCC.

Author details

Guolong Zhang, Peiru Wang and Xiuli Wang*

*Address all correspondence to: wangxiuli20150315@163.com

Institute of Photomedicine, Shanghai Skin Disease Hospital, Tongji University School of Medicine, Shanghai, China

References

[1] Silver FH, Siperko LM, Seehra GP. Mechanobiology of force transduction in dermal tissue. Skin Research and Technology. 2003;**9**(1):3-23

[2] Uitto J. Connective tissue biochemistry of the aging dermis. Age-associated alterations in collagen and elastin. Clinics in Geriatric Medicine. 1989;**5**(1):127-147

[3] Quan T, Fisher GJ. Role of age-associated alterations of the dermal extracellular matrix microenvironment in human skin aging: A mini-review. Gerontology. 2015;**61**(5):427-434. DOI: 10.1159/000371708

[4] Nagase H, Visse R, Murphy G. Structure and function of matrix metalloproteinases and TIMPs. Carvascular Research. 2006;**69**(3):562-573. DOI: 10.1016/j.carres.2005.12.002

[5] Azevedo A, Prado AF, Antonio RC, Issa JP, Gerlach RF, et al. Basic & Clinical Pharmacology & Toxicology. 2014;**115**(4):301-314. DOI: 10.1111/bcpt.12282

[6] Kahari VM, Saarialho-Kere U. Matrix metalloproteinases in skin. Experimental Dermatology. 1997;**6**(5):199-213

[7] McGowan KA, Bauer EA, Smith LT. Localization of type I human skin collagenase in developing embryonic and fetal skin. The Journal of Investigative Dermatology. 1994;**102**(6):951-957

[8] Saarialho-Kere UK, Chang ES, Welgus HG, Parks WC. Distinct localization of collagenase and tissue inhibitor of metalloproteinases expression in wound healing associated with ulcerative pyogenic granuloma. Journal of Clinical Investigation. 1992;**90**(5):1952-1957. DOI: 10.1172/JCI116073

[9] Karelina TV, Goldberg GI, Eisen AZ. Matrilysin (PUMP) correlates with dermal invasion during appendageal development and cutaneous neoplasia. The Journal of Investigative Dermatology. 1994;**103**(4):482-487

[10] Karelina TV, Hruza GJ, Goldberg GI, Eisen AZ. Localization of 92-kDa type IV collagenase in human skin tumors: Comparison with normal human fetal and adult skin. The Journal of Investigative Dermatology. 1993;**100**(2):159-165

[11] Saarialho-Kere UK, Pentland AP, Birkedal-Hansen H, Parks WC, Welgus HG. Distinct populations of basal keratinocytes express stromelysin-1 and stromelysin-2 in chronic wounds. Journal of Clinical Investigation. 1994;**94**(1):79-88. DOI: 10.1172/JCI117351

[12] Zigrino P, Brinckmann J, Niehoff A, Lu Y, Giebeler N, Eckes B, et al. Fibroblast-derived MMP-14 regulates collagen homeostasis in adult skin. Journal of Investigative Dermatology. 2016;**136**(8):1575-1583. DOI: 10.1016/j.jid.2016.03.036

[13] Boyd S, Virolainen S, Parssinen J, Skoog T, van Hogerlinden M, Latonen L, et al. MMP-10 (Stromelysin-2) and MMP-21 in human and murine squamous cell cancer. Experimental Dermatology. 2009; **18**(12): 1044-1052. 10.1111/j.1600-0625.2009.00901.x.

[14] Stenn KS, Paus R. Controls of hair follicle cycling. Physiological Reviews. 2001;**81**(1): 449-494

[15] Hou C, Miao Y, Wang X, Chen C, Lin B, Hu Z. Expression of matrix metalloproteinases and tissue inhibitor of matrix metalloproteinases in the hair cycle. Experimental and Therapeutic Medicine. 2016;**12**(1):231-237. DOI: 10.3892/etm.2016.3319

[16] Yamazaki M, Tsuboi R, Lee YR, Ishidoh K, Mitsui S, Ogawa H. Hair cycle-dependent expression of hepatocyte growth factor (HGF) activator, other proteinases, and proteinase inhibitors correlates with the expression of HGF in rat hair follicles. The Journal of Investigative Dermatology Symposium Proceedings. 1999;**4**(3):312-315

[17] Jarrousse F, Boisnic S, Branchet MC, Beranger JY, Godeau G, Breton L, et al. Identification of clustered cells in human hair follicle responsible for MMP-9 gelatinolytic activity: Consequences for the regulation of hair growth. International Journal of Dermatology. 2001;**40**(6):385-392

[18] Hou C, Miao Y, Wang J, Wang X, Chen CY, Hu ZQ. Collagenase IV plays an important role in regulating hair cycle by inducing VEGF, IGF-1, and TGF-beta expression. Drug Design, Development and Therapy. 2015;**9**:5373-5383. DOI: 10.2147/DDDT.S8912, 10.2147/DDDT.S89124

[19] Saarialho-Kere UK, Kovacs SO, Pentland AP, Olerud JE, Welgus HG, Parks WC. Cell-matrix interactions modulate interstitial collagenase expression by human keratinocytes actively involved in wound healing. Journal of Clinical Investigation. 1993;**92**(6):2858-2866. DOI: 10.1172/JCI116906

[20] Pilcher BK, Dumin J, Schwartz MJ, Mast BA, Schultz GS, Parks WC, et al. Keratinocyte collagenase-1 expression requires an epidermal growth factor receptor autocrine mechanism. The Journal of Biological Chemistry. 1999;**274**(15):10372-10381

[21] Mauviel A, Chen YQ, Kahari VM, Ledo I, Wu M, Rudnicka L, et al. Human recombinant interleukin-1 beta up-regulates elastin gene expression in dermal fibroblasts. Evidence for transcriptional regulation in vitro and in vivo. The Journal of Biological Chemistry. 1993;**268**(9):6520-6524

[22] Salo T, Makela M, Kylmaniemi M, Autio-Harmainen H, Larjava H. Expression of matrix metalloproteinase-2 and -9 during early human wound healing. Laboratory Investigation. 1994;**70**(2):176-182

[23] Lechapt-Zalcman E, Pruliere-Escabasse V, Advenier D, Galiacy S, Charriere-Bertrand C, Coste A, et al. Transforming growth factor-beta1 increases airway wound repair via MMP-2 upregulation: a new pathway for epithelial wound repair? American Journal of Physiology – Lung Cellular and Molecular Physiology. 2006;**290**(6):L1277-L1282. DOI: 10.1152/ajplung.00149.2005

[24] Hattori N, Mochizuki S, Kishi K, Nakajima T, Takaishi H, D'Armiento J, et al. MMP-13 plays a role in keratinocyte migration, angiogenesis, and contraction in mouse skin wound healing. The American Journal of Pathology. 2009;**175**(2):533-546. DOI: 10.2353/ajpath.2009.081080

[25] Rechardt O, Elomaa O, Vaalamo M, Paakkonen K, Jahkola T, Hook-Nikanne J, et al. Stromelysin-2 is upregulated during normal wound repair and is induced by cytokines. Journal of Investigative Dermatology. 2000;**115**(5):778-787. DOI: 10.1046/j.1523-1747.2000.00135.x

[26] Strongin AY, Collier I, Bannikov G, Marmer BL, Grant GA, Goldberg GI. Mechanism of cell surface activation of 72-kDa type IV collagenase. Isolation of the activated form of the membrane metalloprotease. The Journal of Biological Chemistry. 1995;**270**(10):5331-5338

[27] Atkinson JJ, Toennies HM, Holmbeck K, Senior RM. Membrane type 1 matrix metalloproteinase is necessary for distal airway epithelial repair and keratinocyte growth factor receptor expression after acute injury. American Journal of Physiology-Lung Cellular and Molecular Physiology. 2007;**293**(3):L600-L610. DOI: 10.1152/ajplung.00028.2007

[28] Kajita M, Itoh Y, Chiba T, Mori H, Okada A, Kinoh H, et al. Membrane-type 1 matrix metalloproteinase cleaves CD44 and promotes cell migration. The Journal of Cell Biology. 2001;**153**(5):893-904

[29] Endo K, Takino T, Miyamori H, Kinsen H, Yoshizaki T, Furukawa M, et al. Cleavage of syndecan-1 by membrane type matrix metalloproteinase-1 stimulates cell migration. Journal of Biological Chemistry. 2003;**278**(42):40764-40770. DOI: 10.1074/jbc.M306736200

[30] Hasty KA, Hibbs MS, Kang AH, Mainardi CL. Secreted forms of human neutrophil collagenase. The Journal of Biological Chemistry. 1986;**261**(12):5645-5650

[31] Gutierrez-Fernandez A, Inada M, Balbin M, Fueyo A, Pitiot AS, Astudillo A, et al. Increased inflammation delays wound healing in mice deficient in collagenase-2 (MMP-8). FASEB Journal. 2007;**21**(10):2580-2591. DOI: 10.1096/fj.06-7860com

[32] Madlener M, Parks WC, Werner S. Matrix metalloproteinases (MMPs) and their physiological inhibitors (TIMPs) are differentially expressed during excisional skin wound repair. Experimental Cell Research. 1998;**242**(1):201-210. DOI: 10.1006/excr.1998.4049

[33] Cornelius LA, Nehring LC, Harding E, Bolanowski M, Welgus HG, Kobayashi DK, et al. Matrix metalloproteinases generate angiostatin: Effects on neovascularization. Journal of Immunology. 1998;**161**(12):6845-6852

[34] Juncker-Jensen A, Lund LR. Phenotypic overlap between MMP-13 and the plasminogen activation system during wound healing in mice. PLoS One. 2011;**6**(2):e16954. DOI: 10.1371/journal.pone.0016954

[35] Hieta N, Impola U, Lopez-Otin C, Saarialho-Kere U, Kahari VM. Matrix metalloproteinase-19 expression in dermal wounds and by fibroblasts in culture. Journal of Investigative Dermatology. 2003;**121**(5):997-1004. DOI: 10.1046/j.1523-1747.2003.12533.x

[36] Sadowski T, Dietrich S, Koschinsky F, Sedlacek R. Matrix metalloproteinase 19 regulates insulin-like growth factor-mediated proliferation, migration, and adhesion in human keratinocytes through proteolysis of insulin-like growth factor binding protein-3. Molecular Biology of the Cell. 2003;**14**(11):4569-4580. DOI: 10.1091/mbc.E03-01-0009

[37] Ahokas K, Skoog T, Suomela S, Jeskanen L, Impola U, Isaka K, et al. Matrilysin-2 (matrix metalloproteinase-26) is upregulated in keratinocytes during wound repair and early skin carcinogenesis. Journal of Investigative Dermatology. 2005;**124**(4):849-856. DOI: 10.1111/j.0022-202X.2005.23640.x

[38] Saarialho-Kere U, Kerkela E, Jahkola T, Suomela S, Keski-Oja J, Lohi J. Epilysin (MMP-28) expression is associated with cell proliferation during epithelial repair. Journal of Investigative Dermatology. 2002;**119**(1):14-21. DOI: 10.1046/j.1523-1747.2002.01790.x

[39] Krutmann J. Ultraviolet A radiation-induced biological effects in human skin: Relevance for photoaging and photodermatosis. Journal of Dermatological Science. 2000;**23**(Suppl 1): S22-S26

[40] Varani J, Warner RL, Gharaee-Kermani M, Phan SH, Kang S, Chung JH, et al. Vitamin A antagonizes decreased cell growth and elevated collagen-degrading matrix metalloproteinases and stimulates collagen accumulation in naturally aged human skin. Journal of Investigative Dermatology. 2000;**114**(3):480-486. DOI: 10.1046/j.1523-1747.2000.00902.x

[41] Quan T, Qin Z, Xia W, Shao Y, Voorhees JJ, Fisher GJ. Matrix-degrading metalloproteinases in photoaging. Journal of Investigative Dermatology Symposium Proceedings. 2009;**14**(1):20-24. DOI: 10.1038/jidsymp.2009.8

[42] Ham SA, Kang ES, Lee H, Hwang JS, Yoo T, Paek KS, et al. PPARdelta inhibits UVB-induced secretion of MMP-1 through MKP-7-mediated suppression of JNK signaling. Journal of Investigative Dermatology. 2013;**133**(11):2593-2600. DOI: 10.1038/jid.2013.202

[43] Fagot D, Asselineau D, Bernerd F. Matrix metalloproteinase-1 production observed after solar-simulated radiation exposure is assumed by dermal fibroblasts but involves a paracrine activation through epidermal keratinocytes. Photochemistry and Photobiology. 2004;**79**(6):499-505

[44] Fisher GJ, Voorhees JJ. Molecular mechanisms of photoaging and its prevention by retinoic acid: Ultraviolet irradiation induces MAP kinase signal transduction cascades that induce Ap-1-regulated matrix metalloproteinases that degrade human skin in vivo. The Journal of Investigative Dermatology Symposium Proceedings. 1998;**3**(1):61-68

[45] Fisher GJ, Choi HC, Bata-Csorgo Z, Shao Y, Datta S, Wang ZQ, et al. Ultraviolet irradiation increases matrix metalloproteinase-8 protein in human skin in vivo. Journal of Investigative Dermatology. 2001;**117**(2):219-226. DOI: 10.1046/j.0022-202x.2001.01432.x

[46] Rijken F, Kiekens RC, van den Worm E, Lee PL, van Weelden H, Bruijnzeel PL. Pathophysiology of photoaging of human skin: Focus on neutrophils. Photochemical & Photobiological Sciences. 2006;**5**(2):184-189. 10.1039/b502522b.

[47] Chung JH, Seo JY, Lee MK, Eun HC, Lee JH, Kang S, et al. Ultraviolet modulation of human macrophage metalloelastase in human skin in vivo. Journal of Investigative Dermatology. 2002;**119**(2):507-512. DOI: 10.1046/j.1523-1747.2002.01844.x

[48] Tewari A, Grys K, Kollet J, Sarkany R, Young AR. Upregulation of MMP12 and its activity by UVA1 in human skin: Potential implications for photoaging. Journal of Investigative Dermatology. 2014;**134**(10):2598-2609. DOI: 10.1038/jid.2014.173

[49] Fisher GJ, Quan T, Purohit T, Shao Y, Cho MK, He T, et al. Collagen fragmentation promotes oxidative stress and elevates matrix metalloproteinase-1 in fibroblasts in aged human skin. The American Journal of Pathology. 2009;**174**(1):101-114. DOI: 10.2353/ajpath.2009.080599

[50] Hensley K, Floyd RA. Reactive oxygen species and protein oxidation in aging: A look back, a look ahead. Archives of Biochemistry and Biophysics. 2002;**397**(2):377-383. DOI: 10.1006/abbi.2001.2630

[51] Varani J, Dame MK, Rittie L, Fligiel SE, Kang S, Fisher GJ, et al. Decreased collagen production in chronologically aged skin: Roles of age-dependent alteration in fibroblast function and defective mechanical stimulation. The American Journal of Pathology. 2006;**168**(6):1861-1868. DOI: 10.2353/ajpath.2006.051302

[52] Li Y, Xia W, Liu Y, Remmer HA, Voorhees J, Fisher GJ, et al. PLoS One. 2013;**8**(8):e72563. DOI: 10.1371/journal.pone.0072563

[53] Qin Z, Voorhees JJ, Fisher GJ, Quan T. Age-associated reduction of cellular spreading/mechanical force up-regulates matrix metalloproteinase-1 expression and collagen fibril fragmentation via c-Jun/AP-1 in human dermal fibroblasts. Aging Cell. 2014;**13**(6):1028-1037. DOI: 10.1111/acel.12265

[54] Li Y, Lei D, Swindell WR, Xia W, Weng S, Fu J, et al. Age-associated increase in skin fibroblast-derived prostaglandin E2 contributes to reduced collagen levels in elderly human skin. Journal of Investigative Dermatology. 2015;**135**(9):2181-2188. DOI: 10.1038/jid.2015.157

[55] Wang F, Garza LA, Kang S, Varani J, Orringer JS, Fisher GJ, et al. In vivo stimulation of de novo collagen production caused by cross-linked hyaluronic acid dermal filler injections in photodamaged human skin. Archives of Dermatology. 2007;**143**(2):155-163. DOI: 10.1001/archderm.143.2.155

[56] Fisher GJ, Datta SC, Talwar HS, Wang ZQ, Varani J, Kang S, et al. Molecular basis of sun-induced premature skin ageing and retinoid antagonism. Nature. 1996;**379**(6563):335-339. DOI: 10.1038/379335a0

[57] Soter NA. Acute effects of ultraviolet radiation on the skin. Seminars in Dermatology. 1990;**9**(1):11-15

[58] Kutting B, Drexler H. Evaluation of skin-protective means against acute and chronic effects of ultraviolet radiation from sunlight. Current Problems in Dermatology. 2007;**34**:87-97. DOI: 10.1159/000099606

[59] Rijken F, Kiekens RC, Bruijnzeel PL. Skin-infiltrating neutrophils following exposure to solar-simulated radiation could play an important role in photoageing of human skin. British Journal of Dermatology. 2005;**152**(2):321-328. DOI: 10.1111/j.1365-2133.2004.06335.x

[60] Sudel KM, Venzke K, Knussmann-Hartig E, Moll I, Stab F, Wenck H, et al. Tight control of matrix metalloproteinase-1 activity in human skin. Photochemistry and Photobiology. 2003;**78**(4):355-360

[61] Sbardella D, Fasciglione GF, Gioia M, Ciaccio C, Tundo GR, Marini S, et al. Human matrix metalloproteinases: An ubiquitarian class of enzymes involved in several pathological processes. Molecular Aspects of Medicine. 2012;**33**(2):119-208. DOI: 10.1016/j.mam.2011.10.015

[62] Brennan M, Bhatti H, Nerusu KC, Bhagavathula N, Kang S, Fisher GJ, et al. Matrix metalloproteinase-1 is the major collagenolytic enzyme responsible for collagen damage in UV-irradiated human skin. Photochemistry and Photobiology. 2003;**78**(1):43-48

[63] Son WC, Yun JW, Kim BH. Adipose-derived mesenchymal stem cells reduce MMP-1 expression in UV-irradiated human dermal fibroblasts: Therapeutic potential in skin wrinkling. Bioscience, Biotechnology, and Biochemistry. 2015;**79**(6):919-925. DOI: 10.1080/09168451.2015.1008972

[64] Yao C, Lee DH, Oh JH, Kim MK, Kim KH, Park CH, et al. Poly(I:C) induces expressions of MMP-1, −2, and −3 through various signaling pathways including IRF3 in human skin fibroblasts. Journal of Dermatological Science. 2015;**80**(1):54-60. DOI: 10.1016/j.jdermsci.2015.06.017

[65] Wertz K, Seifert N, Hunziker PB, Riss G, Wyss A, Lankin C, et al. Beta-carotene inhibits UVA-induced matrix metalloprotease 1 and 10 expression in keratinocytes by a singlet oxygen-dependent mechanism. Free Radic Biol Med. 2004;**37**(5):654-670. DOI: 10.1016/j.freeradbiomed.2004.05.018.

[66] Vayalil PK, Mittal A, Hara Y, Elmets CA, Katiyar SK. Green tea polyphenols prevent ultraviolet light-induced oxidative damage and matrix metalloproteinases expression in mouse skin. Journal of Investigative Dermatology. 2004;**122**(6):1480-1487. DOI: 10.1111/j.0022-202X.2004.22622.x

[67] Kim HS, Song JH, Youn UJ, Hyun JW, Jeong WS, Lee MY, et al. Inhibition of UVB-induced wrinkle formation and MMP-9 expression by mangiferin isolated from *Anemarrhena asphodeloides*. European Journal of Pharmacology. 2012;**689**(1-3):38-44. DOI: 10.1016/j.ejphar.2012.05.050

[68] Taddese S, Weiss AS, Neubert RH, Schmelzer CE. Mapping of macrophage elastase cleavage sites in insoluble human skin elastin. Matrix Biology. 2008;**27**(5):420-428. DOI: 10.1016/j.matbio.2008.02.001

[69] Taddese S, Weiss AS, Jahreis G, Neubert RH, Schmelzer CE. In vitro degradation of human tropoelastin by MMP-12 and the generation of matrikines from domain 24. Matrix Biology. 2009;**28**(2):84-91. DOI: 10.1016/j.matbio.2008.12.002

[70] Fortino V, Maioli E, Torricelli C, Davis P, Valacchi G. Cutaneous MMPs are differently modulated by environmental stressors in old and young mice. Toxicology Letters. 2007;**173**(2):73-79. DOI: 10.1016/j.toxlet.2007.06.004

[71] Lahmann C, Bergemann J, Harrison G, Young AR. Matrix metalloproteinase-1 and skin ageing in smokers. Lancet. 2001;**357**(9260):935-936. DOI: 10.1016/S0140-6736(00)04220-3

[72] Kobayashi Y. Langerhans' cells produce type IV collagenase (MMP-9) following epicutaneous stimulation with haptens. Immunology. 1997;**90**(4):496-501

[73] Ra HJ, Parks WC, Control of matrix metalloproteinase catalytic activity. Matrix Biology. 2007;**26**(8):587-596. DOI: 10.1016/j.matbio.2007.07.001

[74] Yan C, Boyd DD. Regulation of matrix metalloproteinase gene expression. Journal of Cellular Physiology. 2007;**211**(1):19-26. DOI: 10.1002/jcp.20948

[75] Chiang HM, Lin TJ, Chiu CY, Chang CW, Hsu KC, Fan PC, et al. *Coffea arabica* extract and its constituents prevent photoaging by suppressing MMPs expression and MAP kinase pathway. Food and Chemical Toxicology. 2011;**49**(1):309-318. DOI: 10.1016/j.fct.2010.10.034

[76] Nakajima H, Ezaki Y, Nagai T, Yoshioka R, Imokawa G. Epithelial-mesenchymal interaction during UVB-induced up-regulation of neutral endopeptidase. Biochemical Journal. 2012;**443**(1):297-305. DOI: 10.1042/BJ20111876

[77] Sun ZW, Hwang E, Lee HJ, Lee TY, Song HG, Park SY, et al. Effects of *Galla chinensis* extracts on UVB-irradiated MMP-1 production in hairless mice. Journal of Natural Medicines. 2015;**69**(1):22-34. DOI: 10.1007/s11418-014-0856-6

[78] Wen KC, Fan PC, Tsai SY, Shih IC, Chiang HM. *Ixora parviflora* protects against UVB-induced photoaging by inhibiting the expression of MMPs, MAP kinases, and COX-2 and by promoting type i procollagen synthesis. Evidence-Based Complementary and Alternative Medicine. 2012;**2012**:417346. DOI: 10.1155/2012/417346

[79] Kligman AM, Leyden JJ. Treatment of photoaged skin with topical tretinoin. Skin Pharmacology. 1993;**6**(Suppl 1):78-82

[80] Kligman AM, Dogadkina D, Lavker RM. Effects of topical tretinoin on non-sun-exposed protected skin of the elderly. Journal of the American Academy of Dermatology. 1993;**29**(1):25-33

[81] Gurkan A, Cinarcik S, Huseyinov A. Adjunctive subantimicrobial dose doxycycline: Effect on clinical parameters and gingival crevicular fluid transforming growth factor-beta levels in severe, generalized chronic periodontitis. Journal of Clinical Periodontology. 2005;**32**(3):244-253. DOI: 10.1111/j.1600-051X.2005.00663.x

[82] Paixao-Cavalcante D, van den Berg CW, Goncalves-de-Andrade RM, Fernandes-Pedrosa Mde F, Okamoto CK, Tambourgi DV. Tetracycline protects against dermonecrosis induced by Loxosceles spider venom. Journal of Investigative Dermatology. 2007; **127**(6):1410-1418. 10.1038/sj.jid.5700688.

[83] Apalla Z, Nashan D, Weller RB, Castellsague X. Skin cancer: epidemiology, disease burden, pathophysiology, diagnosis, and therapeutic approaches. Dermatology and Therapy (Heidelb). 2017;**7**(Suppl 1):5-19. DOI: 10.1007/s13555-016-0165-y

[84] Hernandez-Perez M, Mahalingam M. Matrix metalloproteinases in health and disease: Insights from dermatopathology. American Journal of Dermatopathology. 2012;**34**(6): 565-579. DOI: 10.1097/DAD.0b013e31821e8744

[85] Wick MR. Cutaneous melanoma: A current overview. Seminars in Diagnostic Pathology. 2016;**33**(4):225-241. DOI: 10.1053/j.semdp.2016.04.007

[86] Woolley DE, Grafton CA. Collagenase immunolocalization studies of cutaneous secondary melanomas. British Journal of Cancer. 1980;**42**(2):260-265

[87] Boire A, Covic L, Agarwal A, Jacques S, Sherifi S, Kuliopulos A. PAR1 is a matrix metalloprotease-1 receptor that promotes invasion and tumorigenesis of breast cancer cells. Cell. 2005;**120**(3):303-313. DOI: 10.1016/j.cell.2004.12.018

[88] Airola K, Karonen T, Vaalamo M, Lehti K, Lohi J, Kariniemi AL, et al. Expression of collagenases-1 and -3 and their inhibitors TIMP-1 and -3 correlates with the level of invasion in malignant melanomas. British Journal of Cancer. 1999;**80**(5-6):733-743. DOI: 10.1038/sj.bjc.6690417

[89] Montgomery AM, De Clerck YA, Langley KE, Reisfeld RA, Mueller BM. Melanoma-mediated dissolution of extracellular matrix: contribution of urokinase-dependent and metalloproteinase-dependent proteolytic pathways. Cancer Research. 1993;**53**(3):693-700

[90] Blackburn JS, Rhodes CH, Coon CI, Brinckerhoff CE. RNA interference inhibition of matrix metalloproteinase-1 prevents melanoma metastasis by reducing tumor collagenase activity and angiogenesis. Cancer Research. 2007;**67**(22):10849-10858. DOI: 10.1158/0008-5472.CAN-07-1791

[91] Rutter JL, Mitchell TI, Buttice G, Meyers J, Gusella JF, Ozelius LJ, et al. A single nucleotide polymorphism in the matrix metalloproteinase-1 promoter creates an Ets binding site and augments transcription. Cancer Research. 1998;**58**(23):5321-5325

[92] Ye S, Dhillon S, Turner SJ, Bateman AC, Theaker JM, Pickering RM, et al. Invasiveness of cutaneous malignant melanoma is influenced by matrix metalloproteinase 1 gene polymorphism. Cancer Research. 2001;**61**(4):1296-1298

[93] Pearce EG, Laxton RC, Pereira AC, Ye S. Haplotype effects on matrix metalloproteinase-1 gene promoter activity in cancer cells. Molecular Cancer Research. 2007;**5**(3):221-227. DOI: 10.1158/1541-7786.MCR-06-0139

[94] Liu H, Wei Q, Gershenwald JE, Prieto VG, Lee JE, Duvic M, et al. Influence of single nucleotide polymorphisms in the MMP1 promoter region on cutaneous melanoma progression. Melanoma Research. 2012;**22**(2):169-175. DOI: 10.1097/CMR.0b013e32834fc46b

[95] Wang LE, Huang YJ, Yin M, Gershenwald JE, Prieto VG, Lee JE, et al. Promoter polymorphisms in matrix metallopeptidase 1 and risk of cutaneous melanoma. European Journal of Cancer. 2011;**47**(1):107-115. DOI: 10.1016/j.ejca.2010.06.129

[96] Moro N, Mauch C, Zigrino P. Metalloproteinases in melanoma. European Journal of Cell Biology. 2014;**93**(1-2):23-29. DOI: 10.1016/j.ejcb.2014.01.002

[97] Nikkola J, Vihinen P, Vlaykova T, Hahka-Kemppinen M, Kahari VM, Pyrhonen S. High expression levels of collagenase-1 and stromelysin-1 correlate with shorter disease-free survival in human metastatic melanoma. International Journal of Cancer. 2002;**97**(4):432-438

[98] Nikkola J, Vihinen P, Vlaykova T, Hahka-Kemppinen M, Kahari VM, Pyrhonen S. High collagenase-1 expression correlates with a favourable chemoimmunotherapy response in human metastatic melanoma. Melanoma Research. 2001;**11**(2):157-166

[99] Giambernardi TA, Grant GM, Taylor GP, Hay RJ, Maher VM, McCormick JJ, et al. Overview of matrix metalloproteinase expression in cultured human cells. Matrix Biology. 1998;**16**(8):483-496

[100] Giambernardi TA, Sakaguchi AY, Gluhak J, Pavlin D, Troyer DA, Das G, et al. Neutrophil collagenase (MMP-8) is expressed during early development in neural crest cells as well as in adult melanoma cells. Matrix Biology. 2001;**20**(8):577-587

[101] Gutierrez-Fernandez A, Fueyo A, Folgueras AR, Garabaya C, Pennington CJ, Pilgrim S, et al. Matrix metalloproteinase-8 functions as a metastasis suppressor through modulation of tumor cell adhesion and invasion. Cancer Research. 2008;**68**(8):2755-2763. DOI: 10.1158/0008-5472.CAN-07-5154

[102] Palavalli LH, Prickett TD, Wunderlich JR, Wei X, Burrell AS, Porter-Gill P, et al. Analysis of the matrix metalloproteinase family reveals that MMP8 is often mutated in melanoma. Nature Genetics. 2009;**41**(5):518-520. DOI: 10.1038/ng.340

[103] Debniak T, Jakubowska A, Serrano-Fernandez P, Kurzawski G, Cybulski C, Chauhan SR, et al. Association of MMP8 gene variation with an increased risk of malignant melanoma. Melanoma Research. 2011;**21**(5):464-468. DOI: 10.1097/CMR.0b013e3283485fdd

[104] Vihinen P, Koskivuo I, Syrjanen K, Tervahartiala T, Sorsa T, Pyrhonen S. Serum matrix metalloproteinase-8 is associated with ulceration and vascular invasion of malignant melanoma. Melanoma Research. 2008;**18**(4):268-273. DOI: 10.1097/CMR.0b013e3283090031

[105] Vihinen P, Tervahartiala T, Sorsa T, Hansson J, Bastholt L, Aamdal S, et al. Benefit of adjuvant interferon alfa-2b (IFN-alpha) therapy in melanoma patients with high serum MMP-8 levels. Cancer Immunology, Immunotherapy. 2015;**64**(2):173-180. DOI: 10.1007/s00262-014-1620-1

[106] Prosvicova J, Grim J, Kopecky J, Priester P, Slanska I, Trojanova P, et al. Non-specific immunotherapy inhibits angiogenesis – results of the monitoring of serum levels of vascular endothelial growth factor and matrix metalloproteinase 8 in patients with malignant melanoma receiving adjuvant high-dose interferon therapy. Epidemiologie, Mikrobiologie, Imunologie. 2017;**66**(1):15-23

[107] Bodey B, Bodey B Jr, Siegel SE, Kaiser HE. Matrix metalloproteinase expression in malignant melanomas: Tumor-extracellular matrix interactions in invasion and metastasis. In Vivo. 2001;**15**(1):57-64

[108] Corte MD, Gonzalez LO, Corte MG, Quintela I, Pidal I, Bongera M, et al. Collagenase-3 (MMP-13) expression in cutaneous malignant melanoma. The International Journal of Biological Markers. 2005;**20**(4):242-248

[109] Meierjohann S, Hufnagel A, Wende E, Kleinschmidt MA, Wolf K, Friedl P, et al. MMP13 mediates cell cycle progression in melanocytes and melanoma cells: In vitro studies of migration and proliferation. Molecular Cancer. 2010;**9**:201. DOI: 10.1186/1476-4598-9-201

[110] Zigrino P, Kuhn I, Bauerle T, Zamek J, Fox JW, Neumann S, et al. Stromal expression of MMP-13 is required for melanoma invasion and metastasis. Journal of Investigative Dermatology. 2009;**129**(11):2686-2693. DOI: 10.1038/jid.2009.130

[111] Zhao X, Sun B, Li Y, Liu Y, Zhang D, Wang X, et al. Dual effects of collagenase-3 on melanoma: metastasis promotion and disruption of vasculogenic mimicry. Oncotarget. 2015;**6**(11):8890-8899. DOI: 10.18632/oncotarget.3189

[112] Fukuda H, Mochizuki S, Abe H, Okano HJ, Hara-Miyauchi C, Okano H, et al. Host-derived MMP-13 exhibits a protective role in lung metastasis of melanoma cells by local endostatin production. British Journal of Cancer. 2011;**105**(10):1615-1624. DOI: 10.1038/bjc.2011.431

[113] Aksenenko MB, Kirichenko AK, Ruksha TG. Russian study of morphological prognostic factors characterization in BRAF-mutant cutaneous melanoma. Pathology, Research and Practice. 2015;**211**(7):521-527. DOI: 10.1016/j.prp.2015.03.005

[114] Hofmann UB, Eggert AA, Blass K, Brocker EB, Becker JC. Stromal cells as the major source for matrix metalloproteinase-2 in cutaneous melanoma. Archives of Dermatological Research. 2005;**297**(4):154-160. DOI: 10.1007/s00403-005-0588-2

[115] Kurschat P, Wickenhauser C, Groth W, Krieg T, Mauch C. Identification of activated matrix metalloproteinase-2 (MMP-2) as the main gelatinolytic enzyme in malignant melanoma by in situ zymography. Journal of Pathology. 2002;**197**(2):179-187. DOI: 10.1002/path.1080

[116] Jiao Y, Feng X, Zhan Y, Wang R, Zheng S, Liu W, et al. Matrix metalloproteinase-2 promotes alphavbeta3 integrin-mediated adhesion and migration of human melanoma cells by cleaving fibronectin. PLoS One. 2012;**7**(7):e41591. DOI: 10.1371/journal.pone.0041591

[117] Kamyab-Hesari K, Mohtasham N, Aghazadeh N, Biglarian M, Memar B, Kadeh H. The expression of MMP-2 and Ki-67 in head and neck melanoma, and their correlation with clinic-pathologic indices. Journal of Cancer Research and Therapeutics. 2014;**10**(3):696-700. DOI: 10.4103/0973-1482.138122

[118] Liu F, Gomez Garcia AM, Meyskens Jr FL. NADPH oxidase 1 overexpression enhances invasion via matrix metalloproteinase-2 and epithelial-mesenchymal transition in melanoma cells. Journal of Investigative Dermatology. 2012;**132**(8):2033-2041. DOI: 10.1038/jid.2012.119

[119] Akhavan MM, Karimi M, Ghodrati M, Falahtpishe H. AT1 receptors activation enhances the expression of MMP-2, MMP-13 and VEGF but not MMP-9 in B16F10 melanoma cells. Pakistan Journal of Biological Sciences. 2011;**14**(17):821-830

[120] Prakash M, Kale S, Ghosh I, Kundu GC, Datta K. Hyaluronan-binding protein 1 (HABP1/p32/gC1qR) induces melanoma cell migration and tumor growth by NF-kappa B dependent MMP-2 activation through integrin alpha(v)beta(3) interaction. Cell Signaling. 2011;**23**(10):1563-1577. DOI: 10.1016/j.cellsig.2011.04.009

[121] Philip S, Bulbule A, Kundu GC. Osteopontin stimulates tumor growth and activation of promatrix metalloproteinase-2 through nuclear factor-kappa B-mediated induction of membrane type 1 matrix metalloproteinase in murine melanoma cells. Journal of Biological Chemistry. 2001;**276**(48):44926-44935. DOI: 10.1074/jbc.M103334200

[122] Luca M, Huang S, Gershenwald JE, Singh RK, Reich R, Bar-Eli M. Expression of interleukin-8 by human melanoma cells up-regulates MMP-2 activity and increases tumor growth and metastasis. The American Journal of Pathology. 1997;**151**(4):1105-1113

[123] Ohnishi Y, Tajima S, Ishibashi A. Coordinate expression of membrane type-matrix metalloproteinases-2 and 3 (MT2-MMP and MT3-MMP) and matrix metalloproteinase-2 (MMP-2) in primary and metastatic melanoma cells. European Journal of Dermatology. 2001;**11**(5):420-423

[124] Malaponte G, Zacchia A, Bevelacqua Y, Marconi A, Perrotta R, Mazzarino MC, et al. Co-regulated expression of matrix metalloproteinase-2 and transforming growth factor-beta in melanoma development and progression. Oncology Reports. 2010;**24**(1):81-87

[125] Vuoristo MS, Kellokumpu-Lehtinen P, Parvinen LM, Hahka-Kemppinen M, Korpela M, Kumpulainen E, et al. Serum matrix metalloproteinase-2 as a prognostic marker in advanced cutaneous melanoma. Acta Oncologica. 2000;**39**(7):877-879

[126] Wollina U, Hipler UC, Knoll B, Graefe T, Kaatz M, Kirsch K. Serum matrix metalloproteinase-2 in patients with malignant melanoma. Journal of Cancer Research and Clinical Oncology. 2001;**127**(10):631-635

[127] Cotignola J, Roy P, Patel A, Ishill N, Shah S, Houghton A, et al. Functional polymorphisms in the promoter regions of MMP2 and MMP3 are not associated with melanoma progression. Journal of Negative Results in BioMedicine. 2007;**6**:9. DOI: 10.1186/1477-5751-6-9

[128] Lugowska I, Kowalska M, Fuksiewicz M, Kotowicz B, Mierzejewska E, Kosela-Paterczyk H, et al. Serum markers in early-stage and locally advanced melanoma. Tumor Biology. 2015;**36**(11):8277-8285. DOI: 10.1007/s13277-015-3564-2

[129] Kong L, Fang W, Zhong H, Heng W, Li Y, Wu B. Controlled expression of matrix metalloproteinase 9 promotes expression of invasive phenotype of human melanoma cells. Beijing Da Xue Xue Bao. Yi Xue Ban. 2003;**35**(1):7-11

[130] Hamano Y, Kalluri R. Tumstatin, the NC1 domain of alpha3 chain of type IV collagen, is an endogenous inhibitor of pathological angiogenesis and suppresses tumor growth. Biochemical and Biophysical Research Communications. 2005;**333**(2):292-298. DOI: 10.1016/j.bbrc.2005.05.130

[131] Redondo P, Lloret P, Idoate M, Inoges S. Expression and serum levels of MMP-2 and MMP-9 during human melanoma progression. Clinical and Experimental Dermatology. 2005;**30**(5):541-545. DOI: 10.1111/j.1365-2230.2005.01849.x

[132] Nikkola J, Vihinen P, Vuoristo MS, Kellokumpu-Lehtinen P, Kahari VM, Pyrhonen S. High serum levels of matrix metalloproteinase-9 and matrix metalloproteinase-1 are associated with rapid progression in patients with metastatic melanoma. Clinical Cancer Research. 2005;**11**(14):5158-5166. DOI: 10.1158/1078-0432.CCR-04-2478

[133] Cotignola J, Reva B, Mitra N, Ishill N, Chuai S, Patel A, et al. Matrix metalloproteinase-9 (MMP-9) polymorphisms in patients with cutaneous malignant melanoma. BMC Medical Genetics. 2007;**8**:10. DOI: 10.1186/1471-2350-8-10

[134] Walker RA, Woolley DE. Immunolocalisation studies of matrix metalloproteinases-1, -2 and -3 in human melanoma. Virchows Archiv. 1999;**435**(6):574-579

[135] Tas F, Duranyildiz D, Oguz H, Disci R, Kurul S, Yasasever V, et al. Serum matrix metalloproteinase-3 and tissue inhibitor of metalloproteinase-1 in patients with malignant melanoma. Medical Oncology. 2005;**22**(1):39-44. DOI: 10.1385/MO:22:1:039

[136] Vlaykova T, Kurzawski M, Tacheva T, Dimov D, Gulubova M, Yovchev Y, et al. Investigation of the role of MMP3 –1171insA polymorphism in cutaneous malignant melanoma – a preliminary study. Biotechnology & Biotechnological Equipment. 2014; **28**(5):904-910. DOI: 10.1080/13102818.2014.947694

[137] Wagner SN, Ruhri C, Kunth K, Holecek BU, Goos M, Hofler H, et al. Expression of stromelysin 3 in the stromal elements of human basal cell carcinoma. Diagnostic Molecular Pathology. 1992;**1**(3):200-205

[138] Kawasaki K, Kawakami T, Watabe H, Itoh F, Mizoguchi M, Soma Y. Expression of matrilysin (matrix metalloproteinase-7) in primary cutaneous and metastatic melanoma. British Journal of Dermatology. 2007;**156**(4):613-619. DOI: 10.1111/j.1365-2133.2006.07678.x

[139] Kuivanen T, Ahokas K, Virolainen S, Jahkola T, Holtta E, Saksela O, et al. MMP-21 is upregulated at early stages of melanoma progression but disappears with more aggressive phenotype. Virchows Archiv. 2005;**447**(6):954-960. DOI: 10.1007/s00428-005-0046-8

[140] Zhao YG, Xiao AZ, Ni J, Man YG, Sang QX. Expression of matrix metalloproteinase-26 in multiple human cancer tissues and smooth muscle cells. Ai Zheng. 2009;**28**(11): 1168-1175

[141] Sato H, Takino T, Okada Y, Cao J, Shinagawa A, Yamamoto E, et al. A matrix metalloproteinase expressed on the surface of invasive tumour cells. Nature. 1994;**370**(6484):61-65. DOI: 10.1038/370061a0

[142] Sounni NE, Baramova EN, Munaut C, Maquoi E, Frankenne F, Foidart JM, et al. Expression of membrane type 1 matrix metalloproteinase (MT1-MMP) in A2058 melanoma cells is associated with MMP-2 activation and increased tumor growth and vascularization. International Journal of Cancer. 2002;**98**(1):23-28

[143] Kondratiev S, Gnepp DR, Yakirevich E, Sabo E, Annino DJ, Rebeiz E, et al. Expression and prognostic role of MMP2, MMP9, MMP13, and MMP14 matrix metalloproteinases in sinonasal and oral malignant melanomas. Human Pathology. 2008;**39**(3):337-343. DOI: 10.1016/j.humpath.2007.07.003

[144] Hofmann UB, Westphal JR, Zendman AJ, Becker JC, Ruiter DJ, van Muijen GN. Expression and activation of matrix metalloproteinase-2 (MMP-2) and its co-localization with membrane-type 1 matrix metalloproteinase (MT1-MMP) correlate with melanoma progression. Journal of Pathology. 2000;**191**(3):245-256. 10.1002/1096-9896(2000)9999:9999<::AID-PATH632>3.0.CO;2-#.

[145] Shaverdashvili K, Wong P, Ma J, Zhang K, Osman I, Bedogni B. MT1-MMP modulates melanoma cell dissemination and metastasis through activation of MMP2 and RAC1. Pigment Cell Melanoma Research. 2014;**27**(2):287-296. DOI: 10.1111/pcmr.12201

[146] Ma J, Tang X, Wong P, Jacobs B, Borden EC, Bedogni B. Noncanonical activation of Notch1 protein by membrane type 1 matrix metalloproteinase (MT1-MMP) controls melanoma cell proliferation. Journal of Biological Chemistry. 2014;**289**(12):8442-8449. DOI: 10.1074/jbc.M113.516039

[147] Shaverdashvili K, Zhang K, Osman I, Honda K, Jobava R, Bedogni B. MT1-MMP dependent repression of the tumor suppressor SPRY4 contributes to MT1-MMP driven melanoma cell motility. Oncotarget. 2015;**6**(32):33512-33522. DOI: 10.18632/oncotarget.5258

[148] Marusak C, Bayles I, Ma J, Gooyit M, Gao M, Chang M, et al. The thiirane-based selective MT1-MMP/MMP2 inhibitor ND-322 reduces melanoma tumor growth and delays metastatic dissemination. Pharmacological Research. 2016;**113**(Pt A):515-520. DOI: 10.1016/j.phrs.2016.09.033

[149] Tatti O, Arjama M, Ranki A, Weiss SJ, Keski-Oja J, Lehti K. Membrane-type-3 matrix metalloproteinase (MT3-MMP) functions as a matrix composition-dependent effector of melanoma cell invasion. PLoS One. 2011;**6**(12):e28325. DOI: 10.1371/journal.pone.0028325

[150] Tatti O, Gucciardo E, Pekkonen P, Holopainen T, Louhimo R, Repo P, et al. MMP16 Mediates a Proteolytic Switch to Promote Cell-Cell Adhesion, Collagen Alignment, and Lymphatic Invasion in Melanoma. Cancer Research. 2015;**75**(10):2083-2094. DOI: 10.1158/0008-5472.CAN-14-1923

[151] Zhang Z, Zhu S, Yang Y, Ma X, Guo S. Matrix metalloproteinase-12 expression is increased in cutaneous melanoma and associated with tumor aggressiveness. Tumor Biology. 2015;**36**(11):8593-8600. DOI: 10.1007/s13277-015-3622-9

[152] Muller M, Beck IM, Gadesmann J, Karschuk N, Paschen A, Proksch E, et al. MMP19 is upregulated during melanoma progression and increases invasion of melanoma cells. Modern Pathology. 2010;**23**(4):511-521. DOI: 10.1038/modpathol.2009.183

[153] Moogk D, da Silva IP, Ma MW, Friedman EB, de Miera EV, Darvishian F, et al. Melanoma expression of matrix metalloproteinase-23 is associated with blunted tumor immunity and poor responses to immunotherapy. Journal of Translational Medicine. 2014;**12**:342. 10.1186/s12967-014-0342-7

[154] Verkouteren JA, Ramdas KH, Wakkee M, Nijsten T. Epidemiology of basal cell carcinoma: scholarly review. British Journal of Dermatology. 2017. DOI: 10.1111/bjd.15321

[155] Chu CY, Cha ST, Chang CC, Hsiao CH, Tan CT, Lu YC, et al. Involvement of matrix metalloproteinase-13 in stromal-cell-derived factor 1 alpha-directed invasion of human basal cell carcinoma cells. Oncogene. 2007;**26**(17):2491-2501. DOI: 10.1038/sj.onc.1210040

[156] Oh ST, Kim HS, Yoo NJ, Lee WS, Cho BK, Reichrath J. Increased immunoreactivity of membrane type-1 matrix metalloproteinase (MT1-MMP) and beta-catenin in high-risk basal cell carcinoma. British Journal of Dermatology. 2011;**165**(6):1197-1204. DOI: 10.1111/j.1365-2133.2011.10506.x

[157] Varani J, Hattori Y, Chi Y, Schmidt T, Perone P, Zeigler ME, et al. Collagenolytic and gelatinolytic matrix metalloproteinases and their inhibitors in basal cell carcinoma of skin: comparison with normal skin. British Journal of Cancer. 2000;**82**(3):657-665. DOI: 10.1054/bjoc.1999.0978

[158] Zlatarova ZI, Softova EB, Dokova KG, Messmer EM. Expression of matrix metalloproteinase-1, -9, -13, and tissue inhibitor of metalloproteinases-1 in basal cell carcinomas of the eyelid. Graefes Archive For Clinical And Experimental Ophthalmology. 2012;**250**(3):425-431. DOI: 10.1007/s00417-011-1810-x

[159] Monhian N, Jewett BS, Baker SR, Varani J. Matrix metalloproteinase expression in normal skin associated with basal cell carcinoma and in distal skin from the same patients. Archives of Facial Plastic Surgery. 2005;**7**(4):238-243. DOI: 10.1001/archfaci.7.4.238

[160] Son KD, Kim TJ, Lee YS, Park GS, Han KT, Lim JS, et al. Comparative analysis of immunohistochemical markers with invasiveness and histologic differentiation in squamous cell carcinoma and basal cell carcinoma of the skin. Journal of Surgical Oncology. 2008;**97**(7):615-620. DOI: 10.1002/jso.21006

[161] Vanjaka-Rogosic L, Puizina-Ivic N, Miric L, Rogosic V, Kuzmic-Prusac I, Babic MS, et al. Matrix metalloproteinases and E-cadherin immunoreactivity in different basal cell carcinoma histological types. Acta Histochemica. 2014;**116**(5):688-693. DOI: 10.1016/j.acthis.2013.12.007

[162] Ciurea ME, Cernea D, Georgescu CC, Cotoi OS, Patrascu V, Parvanescu H, et al. Expression of CXCR4, MMP-13 and beta-catenin in different histological subtypes of facial basal cell carcinoma. Romanian Journal of Morphology and Embryology. 2013;**54**(4):939-951

[163] Hattori Y, Nerusu KC, Bhagavathula N, Brennan M, Hattori N, Murphy HS, et al. Vascular expression of matrix metalloproteinase-13 (collagenase-3) in basal cell carcinoma. Experimental and Molecular Pathology. 2003;**74**(3):230-237

[164] Alvarez Suarez ML, Gonzalez Vazquez LO, Barbon Garcia JJ, Vazquez Rojo J, Lamelas Suarez-Pola ML, Vizoso Pineiro FJ. Collagenase-3 (MMP-13) expression in epithelial cancers of the eyelids. Archivos de la Sociedad Española de Oftalmología. 2004;**79**(6):281-288

[165] Gozdzialska A, Wojas-Pelc A, Drag J, Brzewski P, Jaskiewicz J, Pastuszczak M. Expression of metalloproteinases (MMP-2 and MMP-9) in basal-cell carcinoma. Molecular Biology Reports. 2016;**43**(10):1027-1033. DOI: 10.1007/s11033-016-4040-9

[166] Grigioni WF, D'Errico A, Fiorentino M, Baccarini P, Onisto M, Caenazzo C, et al. Gelatinase A (MMP-2) and its mRNA detected in both neoplastic and stromal cells of tumors with different invasive and metastatic properties. Diagnostic Molecular Pathology. 1994;**3**(3):163-169

[167] de Oliveira Poswar F, de Carvalho Fraga CA, Gomes ES, Farias LC, Souza LW, Santos SH, et al. Protein expression of MMP-2 and MT1-MMP in actinic keratosis, squamous cell carcinoma of the skin, and basal cell carcinoma. International Journal of Surgical Pathology. 2015;**23**(1):20-25. 10.1177/1066896914540998

[168] Boyd S, Tolvanen K, Virolainen S, Kuivanen T, Kyllonen L, Saarialho-Kere U. Differential expression of stromal MMP-1, MMP-9 and TIMP-1 in basal cell carcinomas of immunosuppressed patients and controls. Virchows Archiv. 2008;**452**(1):83-90. DOI: 10.1007/s00428-007-0526-0

[169] Kerkela E, Ala-aho R, Lohi J, Grenman R, MK V, Saarialho-Kere U. Differential patterns of stromelysin-2 (MMP-10) and MT1-MMP (MMP-14) expression in epithelial skin cancers. British Journal of Cancer. 2001;**84**(5):659-669. DOI: 10.1054/bjoc.2000.1634

[170] Kadeh H, Saravani S, Heydari F, Shahraki S. Differential immunohistochemical expression of matrix metalloproteinase-10 (MMP-10) in non-melanoma skin cancers of the head and neck. Pathology, Research and Practice. 2016;**212**(10):867-871. DOI: 10.1016/j.prp.2016.06.015

[171] Thewes M, Worret WI, Engst R, Ring J. Stromelysin-3 (ST-3): Immunohistochemical characterization of the matrix metalloproteinase (MMP)-11 in benign and malignant skin tumours and other skin disorders. Clinical and Experimental Dermatology. 1999;**24**(2):122-126

[172] Hartmann-Petersen S, Tammi RH, Tammi MI, Kosma VM. Depletion of cell surface CD44 in nonmelanoma skin tumours is associated with increased expression of matrix metalloproteinase 7. British Journal of Dermatology. 2009;**160**(6):1251-1257. DOI: 10.1111/j.1365-2133.2009.09031.x

[173] Moore MG, Bennett RG. Basal cell carcinoma in asians: a retrospective analysis of ten patients. Journal of Skin Cancer. 2012;**2012**:741397. DOI: 10.1155/2012/741397

[174] Kerkela E, Ala-Aho R, Jeskanen L, Rechardt O, Grenman R, Shapiro SD, et al. Expression of human macrophage metalloelastase (MMP-12) by tumor cells in skin cancer. Journal of Investigative Dermatology. 2000;**114**(6):1113-1119. DOI: 10.1046/j.1523-1747.2000.00993.x

[175] Ahokas K, Lohi J, Illman SA, Llano E, Elomaa O, Impola U, et al. Matrix metalloproteinase-21 is expressed epithelially during development and in cancer and is up-regulated by transforming growth factor-beta1 in keratinocytes. Laboratory Investigation. 2003;**83**(12):1887-1899

[176] Green AC, Olsen CM. Cutaneous squamous cell carcinoma: An epidemiological review. British Journal of Dermatology. 2017. DOI: 10.1111/bjd.15324

[177] Barton V, Armeson K, Hampras S, Ferris LK, Visvanathan K, Rollison D, et al. Nonmelanoma skin cancer and risk of all-cause and cancer-related mortality: A systematic review. Archives of Dermatological Research. 2017;**309**(4):243-251. DOI: 10.1007/s00403-017-1724-5

[178] Tsukifuji R, Tagawa K, Hatamochi A, Shinkai H. Expression of matrix metalloproteinase-1, -2 and -3 in squamous cell carcinoma and actinic keratosis. British Journal of Cancer. 1999;**80**(7):1087-1091. DOI: 10.1038/sj.bjc.6690468

[179] Ramos MC, Steinbrenner H, Stuhlmann D, Sies H, Brenneisen P. Induction of MMP-10 and MMP-1 in a squamous cell carcinoma cell line by ultraviolet radiation. Biological Chemistry. 2004;**385**(1):75-86. DOI: 10.1515/BC.2004.010

[180] Johansson N, Airola K, Grenman R, Kariniemi AL, Saarialho-Kere U, Kahari VM. Expression of collagenase-3 (matrix metalloproteinase-13) in squamous cell carcinomas of the head and neck. The American Journal of Pathology. 1997;**151**(2):499-508

[181] Hata H, Abe R, Suto A, Homma E, Fujita Y, Aoyagi S, et al. MMP13 can be a useful differentiating marker between squamous cell carcinoma and benign hyperkeratotic

lesions in recessive dystrophic epidermolysis bullosa. British Journal of Dermatology. 2015;**172**(3):769-773. 10.1111/bjd.13302.

[182] Lederle W, Hartenstein B, Meides A, Kunzelmann H, Werb Z, Angel P, et al. MMP13 as a stromal mediator in controlling persistent angiogenesis in skin carcinoma. Carcinogenesis. 2010;**31**(7):1175-1184. DOI: 10.1093/carcin/bgp248

[183] Meides A, Gutschalk CM, Devel L, Beau F, Czarny B, Hensler S, et al. Effects of selective MMP-13 inhibition in squamous cell carcinoma depend on estrogen. International Journal of Cancer. 2014;**135**(12):2749-2759. DOI: 10.1002/ijc.28866

[184] Moilanen M, Pirila E, Grenman R, Sorsa T, Salo T. Expression and regulation of collagenase-2 (MMP-8) in head and neck squamous cell carcinomas. Journal of Pathology. 2002;**197**(1):72-81. DOI: 10.1002/path.1078

[185] Ahmed Haji Omar A, Haglund C, Virolainen S, Hayry V, Atula T, Kontio R, et al. MMP-7, MMP-8, and MMP-9 in oral and cutaneous squamous cell carcinomas. Oral Surgery, Oral Medicine, Oral Pathology, Oral Radiology. 2015;**119**(4):459-467. DOI: 10.1016/j.oooo.2014.12.019

[186] Kobayashi T, Onoda N, Takagi T, Hori H, Hattori S, Nagai Y, et al. Immunolocalizations of human gelatinase (type IV collagenase, MMP-9) and TIMP (tissue inhibitor of metalloproteinases) in normal epidermis and some epidermal tumors. Archives of Dermatological Research. 1996;**288**(5-6):239-244

[187] Borchers AH, Steinbauer H, Schafer BS, Kramer M, Bowden GT, Fusenig NE. Fibroblast-directed expression and localization of 92-kDa type IV collagenase along the tumor-stroma interface in an in vitro three-dimensional model of human squamous cell carcinoma. Molecular Carcinogenesis. 1997;**19**(4):258-266

[188] Verdolini R, Amerio P, Goteri G, Bugatti L, Lucarini G, Mannello B, et al. Cutaneous carcinomas and preinvasive neoplastic lesions. Role of MMP-2 and MMP-9 metalloproteinases in neoplastic invasion and their relationship with proliferative activity and p53 expression. Journal of Cutaneous Pathology. 2001;**28**(3):120-126

[189] Poswar FO, Fraga CA, Farias LC, Feltenberger JD, Cruz VP, Santos SH, et al. Immunohistochemical analysis of TIMP-3 and MMP-9 in actinic keratosis, squamous cell carcinoma of the skin, and basal cell carcinoma. Pathology, Research and Practice. 2013;**209**(11):705-709. DOI: 10.1016/j.prp.2013.08.002

[190] Kuivanen T, Jeskanen L, Kyllonen L, Isaka K, Saarialho-Kere U. Matrix metalloproteinase-26 is present more frequently in squamous cell carcinomas of immunosuppressed compared with immunocompetent patients. Journal of Cutaneous Pathology. 2009;**36**(9):929-936. DOI: 10.1111/j.1600-0560.2009.01188.x

[191] Nan H, Niu T, Hunter DJ, Han J. Missense polymorphisms in matrix metalloproteinase genes and skin cancer risk. Cancer Epidemiology, Biomarkers & Prevention. 2008;**17**(12): 3551-3557. DOI: 10.1158/1055-9965.EPI-08-0606

[192] Dumas V, Kanitakis J, Charvat S, Euvrard S, Faure M, Claudy A. Expression of basement membrane antigens and matrix metalloproteinases 2 and 9 in cutaneous basal and squamous cell carcinomas. Anticancer Research. 1999;**19**(4B):2929-2938

[193] O'Grady A, Dunne C, O'Kelly P, Murphy GM, Leader M, Kay E. Differential expression of matrix metalloproteinase (MMP)-2, MMP-9 and tissue inhibitor of metalloproteinase (TIMP)-1 and TIMP-2 in non-melanoma skin cancer: implications for tumour progression. Histopathology. 2007;**51**(6):793-804. DOI: 10.1111/j.1365-2559.2007.02885.x

[194] McCawley LJ, Wright J, LaFleur BJ, Crawford HC, Matrisian LM. Keratinocyte expression of MMP3 enhances differentiation and prevents tumor establishment. The American Journal of Pathology. 2008;**173**(5):1528-1539. DOI: 10.2353/ajpath.2008.080132

[195] Nyman M. Ilska in anesthesia – "continued education should be worthwhile!". Vårdfacket. 1989;**13**(4):17-18

[196] Kivisaari AK, Kallajoki M, Mirtti T, McGrath JA, Bauer JW, Weber F, et al. Transformation-specific matrix metalloproteinases (MMP)-7 and MMP-13 are expressed by tumour cells in epidermolysis bullosa-associated squamous cell carcinomas. British Journal of Dermatology. 2008;**158**(4):778-785. DOI: 10.1111/j.1365-2133.2008.08466.x

[197] Chuang HC, Su CY, Huang HY, Huang CC, Chien CY, Du YY, et al. Active matrix metalloproteinase-7 is associated with invasion in buccal squamous cell carcinoma. Modern Pathology. 2008;**21**(12):1444-1450. DOI: 10.1038/modpathol.2008.99

[198] Mitsui H, Suarez-Farinas M, Gulati N, Shah KR, Cannizzaro MV, Coats I, et al. Gene expression profiling of the leading edge of cutaneous squamous cell carcinoma: IL-24-driven MMP-7. Journal of Investigative Dermatology. 2014;**134**(5):1418-1427. DOI: 10.1038/jid.2013.494

[199] Kivisaari AK, Kallajoki M, Ala-aho R, McGrath JA, Bauer JW, Konigova R, et al. Matrix metalloproteinase-7 activates heparin-binding epidermal growth factor-like growth factor in cutaneous squamous cell carcinoma. British Journal of Dermatology. 2010;**163**(4):726-735. DOI: 10.1111/j.1365-2133.2010.09924.x

[200] Gutschalk CM, Yanamandra AK, Linde N, Meides A, Depner S, Mueller MM. GM-CSF enhances tumor invasion by elevated MMP-2, -9, and -26 expression. Cancer Medicine. 2013;**2**(2):117-129. DOI: 10.1002/cam4.20

[201] Sato T, Iwai M, Sakai T, Sato H, Seiki M, Mori Y, et al. Enhancement of membrane-type 1-matrix metalloproteinase (MT1-MMP) production and sequential activation of progelatinase A on human squamous carcinoma cells co-cultured with human dermal fibroblasts. British Journal of Cancer. 1999;**80**(8):1137-1143. DOI: 10.1038/sj.bjc.6690477

[202] Hernandez-Perez M, El-hajahmad M, Massaro J, Mahalingam M. Expression of gelatinases (MMP-2, MMP-9) and gelatinase activator (MMP-14) in actinic keratosis and in in situ and invasive squamous cell carcinoma. American Journal of Dermatopathology. 2012;**34**(7):723-728. DOI: 10.1097/DAD.0b013e31824b1ddf

[203] Rosenthal EL, McCrory A, Talbert M, Carroll W, Magnuson JS, Peters GE. Expression of proteolytic enzymes in head and neck cancer-associated fibroblasts. Archives of Otolaryngology – Head & Neck Surgery. 2004;**130**(8):943-947. DOI: 10.1001/archotol.130.8.943

[204] Kerkela E, Ala-aho R, Klemi P, Grenman S, Shapiro SD, Kahari VM, et al. Metalloelastase (MMP-12) expression by tumour cells in squamous cell carcinoma of the vulva correlates with invasiveness, while that by macrophages predicts better outcome. Journal of Pathology. 2002;**198**(2):258-269. DOI: 10.1002/path.1198

[205] Impola U, Toriseva M, Suomela S, Jeskanen L, Hieta N, Jahkola T, et al. Matrix metalloproteinase-19 is expressed by proliferating epithelium but disappears with neoplastic dedifferentiation. International Journal of Cancer. 2003;**103**(6):709-716. DOI: 10.1002/ijc.10902

Chapter 7

Matrix Metalloproteinases in Melanoma with and without Regression

Alexandra Bastian, Luciana Nichita and
Sabina Zurac

Additional information is available at the end of the chapter

http://dx.doi.org/10.5772/intechopen.72931

Abstract

Cutaneous melanoma is an aggressive tumor with increasing incidence worldwide. Recent development of promising treatments based on immune checkpoints blockade in cancer immunotherapy or signal transduction inhibitors (B-Raf enzyme inhibitor and MEK inhibitor) requires identification of new biomarkers predictive of either prognosis and/or therapeutic response. Dynamic interaction between melanoma and normal host cells influences tumor progression; proteins regulating connections between melanoma cells and extracellular matrix facilitate tumor invasion and dissemination. We discuss the various functions of matrix metalloproteinases (MMPs) and tissue inhibitors of matrix metalloproteinases (TIMPs) in melanoma and their possible role as prognostic and/or predictive biomarkers. We also studied the correlation with regression of expression of several MMPs and TIMPs in melanoma; regressed and nonregressed components are in fact different tumor subclones; in some cases of melanoma with regression (with a specific morphology), the biologic aggressiveness of the tumor and implicitly the overall prognosis may be more favorable than that of melanoma without regression thus offering the possibility of a supplemental stratification of these patients beyond AJCC staging.

Keywords: melanoma, regression, matrix metalloproteinases, tissue inhibitors of matrix metalloproteinases, biomarkers

1. Introduction

Cutaneous melanoma represents one of the most important challenges in routine dermato-oncologic practice due to its increasing incidence worldwide. Its unfavorable prognosis with the increasing number of annual deaths and impressive death toll even in incipient melanoma cases [1] indicate that current stratification of melanoma patients staging system (American Joint Committee on Cancer—AJCC) based on certain morphologic parameters—Breslow thickness, ulceration, nodal and distant metastases—and a serum one—lactate dehydrogenase, is unsatisfactory for both tumor biologic behavior assessment and predictive value of the systemic treatment [2].

The most problematic melanoma patients fall in two main categories: patients with advanced disease (highly invasive thick lesions and/or regional lymph node metastasis) and patients with progressive disease despite incipient stage.

In case of patients with advanced disease, despite major efforts to improve treatment, no significant advance was obtained in the last two decades; lately, development of promising treatments based on immune checkpoints blockade in cancer immunotherapy (nivolumab and pembrolizumab as PD-1 inhibitors; ipilimumab as anti-CTLA4 monoclonal antibody) or signal transduction inhibitors such as B-Raf enzyme inhibitor (vemurafenib and dabrafenib) and MEK inhibitor (trametinib) has been attained [3–8]. Even so, most patients develop acquired resistance with subsequent evolution *in faust*; potential years of life lost due to cutaneous melanoma remain as an epidemiologic indicator without significant improvement despite the extremely expensive costs of the therapy [9].

The other type of patients, those with progressive disease despite incipient stage belongs to pT1 melanomas (less than 1 mm in maximum thickness, i.e., thin melanomas). Prognosis is highly favorable if the tumor is localized (without metastases, either local or distant), surgical resection with 1 cm healthy tissue being curative but there are few patients that eventually die due to disease progression. For this incipient stage, we must look to the dark side of the statistical data: 5 years survival rate for pT1 melanomas is 97.7% with 2.3% mortality due to disease; 10 years survival rate for pT1 melanomas is 95.1% with 4.9% mortality due to disease [10]. Moreover, in case of patients with even thinner lesions (less than 0.75 mm), 10 years survival rate is 97% with a mortality rate due to disease of 3% [11, 12]. These data highlight the need for a supplementary stratification of patients with thin melanoma in "low risk" and "high risk" groups with subsequent more aggressive therapeutic approach for patients identified as "high risk" [13].

Identification of prognostic and/or predictive biomarkers is particularly difficult in cutaneous melanoma due to its complex biologic evolution, encumbered by myriad of different events caused by deregulations of several pathways [14]. Dynamic interaction between melanoma and normal host cells influences tumor progression; proteins regulating connections between melanoma cells and extracellular matrix facilitate tumor invasion and dissemination [15]. Cell adhesion molecules known to facilitate the metastatic potential of many cancers are also altered in melanoma when progressing from the non-invasive to the invasive growth phase and associate increased melanoma thickness and decreased survival [16, 17].

It becomes an imperious task that enzymes involved in degrading extracellular matrix should be investigated in relation with cancer invasion and metastases; these biomolecules belong to the metalloproteinases group that includes several classes of protease enzymes: matrix metalloproteinases (MMPs), a disintegrin and metalloproteinases (ADAMs) and ADAMs with thrombospondin motifs (ADAMTS). All of them are zinc-containing endopeptidases of metzincins family, some extracellular/soluble (most of MMPs and ADAMTS), the others membrane-bounded biomolecules (membrane-type MMPs (MT-MMPs) and ADAMs).

Matrix metalloproteinases (MMPs) represent a complex family of biomolecules accomplishing a myriad of activities with equally physiological and pathological inferences. MMPs are involved in embryologic development and in wound healing as key players in epithelial to mesenchymal transition by enabling cell-cell detachment with subsequent basement membrane perforation; they also initiate Snail positive mechanisms of MMPs expression stimulation *via* increasing reactive oxygen species production [18–22]. MMPs are classified based on their primary function: collagenases (MMP-1, MMP-8, MMP-13, MMP-18), gelatinases (MMP-2, MMP-9), stromelysins (MMP-3, MMP-10), matrilysins (MMP-7, MMP-26); also, MMPs include six forms of MT-MMPs (four transmembranary proteins of which two are anchored to the membrane *via* glycosylphosphatidylinositol) and a group of seven MMPs (metalloelastase (MMP-12), MMP-19, enamelysin (MMP-20), MMP-22, MMP-23, epilysin (MMP-28)), some with still unknown biological function in humans [23, 24].

MMPs dysfunctions contribute to various diseases: degenerative diseases of the brain, atherosclerosis, aortic aneurysm, arthritis, and cirrhosis [25, 26]. In cancer, MMPs facilitate invasion and metastasis and participate as regulators of tumor cells proliferation and apoptosis; also, they intervene in tumor differentiation, tumor immune-resistance, and tumor angiogenesis [27, 28].

In tumor invasion, they mediate adhesion of tumor cells to extracellular matrix components and concomitant proteolysis of extracellular matrix, thus favoring migration of tumor cells into the areas of matrix degradation [29]. Another important role of MMPs in cancer is represented by creation of a local environment able to host and provide specific conditions required by metastatic cells to survive in a distant organ—"metastatic niche" [30].

MMP-1 is a collagenase correlated with enhanced invasiveness and metastasis in melanoma. It is overexpressed in invasive melanoma comparing with *in situ* or microinvasive melanomas where MMP-1 is absent [31]; its knocking down in melanoma cell line diminished the tumor cell capacities for metastasis after implanting in nude mice [32] and, conversely, its introduction in noninvasive melanoma cells induces a metastatic phenotype *in vivo* [33]. MMP1 production is noticed especially in stromal fibroblasts being also involved in PAR1 thrombin receptor activation with subsequent role in increasing tumor progression and metastatic capability of tumor cells [34–36].

MMP-2 (gelatinase A) has an important role in tumor progression due to its ability to degrade collagen IV present in basement membrane; its presence is of outmost importance for tumor invasion, fact demonstrated by the significant reduction of invasion through basement membrane by treating A2058 melanoma cell line culture with an antibody anti human type-IV collagenase [37]. Moreover, in cell culture, MMP-2 is present as activated biomolecules when highly invasive melanoma cells lines are cultured in collagen lattices; by contrast its activity is inhibited by antibodies against MT1-MMP, TIMP-2, and through MMP-2 cleavage by MT1-MMP [38]. It is expressed in melanomatous cells and stromal cells especially in peritumoral areas where its proteolytic activity is present [39]. Using the B16-melanoma cell line mouse model it was shown that MMP-2 expression was predominantly present at the tumor-stroma border indicating stromal cells as primary source for this protease [40]. In another cell model, using human melanoma cell lines M3 Da and M1Dor cocultured with dermal fibroblasts, it was shown that MMP-2 expression in membrane extracts was enhanced. Since stromal and cancer cell contacts have been shown to occur after disruption of the ECM, it is assumed that fibroblasts may influence melanoma cell invasion after the beginning of tumor progression through the dermis [41]. MMP-2 binds to $\alpha v\beta 3$ integrin and regulates $\alpha v\beta 3$ integrin-dependent tumor cell migration most likely by facilitating $\alpha v\beta 3$ integrin binding to previously cleaved extracellular matrix components; one such component, fibronectin, is cleaved by MMP-2 thus facilitating $\alpha v\beta 3$ integrin binding and subsequently migration of tumor cells [42].

MMP-2 expression is correlated with prognosis being proposed as an independent prognostic factor [43]. MMP-2 expression is variable in melanocytic tumors, according to their biologic aggressiveness. Thus, in benign melanocytic tumors (common nevocellular nevi), junctional nevi and melanoma, MMP-2 is present with differences in number according to cytonuclear and architectural features (more numerous cells as cell atypia and architectural disarray increase) [44–46]; MMP-2 was found over-expressed in lesional keratinocytes and enhanced by UVB-irradiation, but not found in melanocytic cells [47]; moreover, occurring of distant metastases is more frequent in melanomas with MMP-2 overexpression in primary tumor [44] but MMP-2 is not present in metastatic melanoma [43]. Also, due to the relation between p-Akt and MMP2, MMP2 could be used as a predictive biomarker for vemurafenib resistance as vemurafenib-treated patients with overexpression of MMP-2 might be more prone to develop resistance [43, 48].

MMP-3 (stromelysin-1) is a metalloproteinase with double role in tumor development, both in tumor progression and tumor suppressing. It activates MMP-1, thus increasing the invasion capabilities of the tumor cells [49]. MMP-3 is overexpressed in metastases of melanoma and associates significantly shorter disease-free survival than patients with lower levels of MMP-3 expression shorter [50]. Other data show that MMP-3 has antitumor effects in squamous cell carcinoma, thus tumors in mmp3 null mice are more aggressive than in control, most likely due to its pro-apoptotic effect in neoplastic cells [51].

MMP-7 (matrilysin) triggers proteolytic cleavage of HB-EGF, a biomolecule with pro-tumor activity in melanoma by both EGFR ligand role and MAPK and PI3K/Akt pathways activator [52–54]. MMP-7 expression was demonstrated in melanomas both primary (up to 80% of primary tumors) and metastatic ones (all the metastatic tumors) while it was absent in both common and Spitz nevi; MMP-7 was identified in tumor cells (both immunohistochemically and by *in situ* hybridization); Western blotting revealed the presence of active MMP-7 in all melanomas (both primary and metastatic); moreover, the MMP-7 immunohistochemical staining score was correlated with Breslow index (higher the MMP-7 positivity score, higher the Breslow thickness of the tumor) and 5-year survival (100% 5-year survival in case of MMP-7 negative melanomas and significant lower percentage—26.3% 5-year survival in case of MMP-7 positive cases), thus raising the issue of its selection as prognostic marker [55].

MMP-8 is a collagenase with anti-tumor attributes. MMP-8 expression is reverse correlated with metastatic potential of breast cancer tumor cells [56, 57]. Several different stable clones of murine B16F10 melanoma cells (normally MMP-8 negative) transfected with murine MMP-8 cDNA develop significantly less numerous and smaller lung metastases after injection in *Mmp8*$^{-/-}$ C57BL/6 mice strain mice; moreover, these MMP-8+ clones obtained from B16F10 melanoma cells or B16F10 melanoma cells incubated with recombinant MMP-8 showed significant *in vitro* diminishing of invasive abilities compared with B16F10 controls due to increased tumor cells adherence to type I collagen and laminin-1 from extracellular matrix [58]. MMP-8 gene is often mutated in melanoma and MMP8-null mice have significantly increased incidence of skin tumors while bone-marrow transplantation (offering neutrophil-derived MMP8) restore MMP-8 antitumor protection [59, 60]. The antitumor properties of MMP-8 are related rather to its capacity to process proinflammatory biomolecules (MMP-8 absence allows the development of an important inflammatory response elicited by chemical substances with carcinogenetic properties) than to its collagenase function [61].

MMP-9 (gelatinase B), similar to MMP-2, is present in melanoma both in tumor cells and stroma with enhance activity at tumor border [39]. However, by contrast to MMP-2 that has tumor progression effects, MMP-9 has dual role, in some cases with anti-tumor activities. Evidences of such effects are both experimental demonstrated as HPV16 related carcinomas have more aggressive biologic behavior in mmp-9 null mice [62], and clinical confirmed as MMP-9 overexpression in colonic and breast carcinoma bears a positive significance—more favorable prognosis [63, 64]. A mechanism for tumor suppressing activity may be represented by inhibition of angiogenesis; collagen IV degradation by MMP-9 releases tumstatin, a biomolecule that inhibits endothelial cells activity and subsequently tumor angiogenesis [65, 66].

MMP-10 (stromelysin-2) over-expression in melanoma was recorded mainly in the extracellular matrix, adjacent both tumor cells and blood vessels, being more likely involved in tumor growth [67]. Its expression is rapidly increased after UV exposure in SCL-1 squamous cell carcinoma cell line [68] is present in stromal cells in squamous cell carcinoma [69] and it seems to be correlated with unfavorable prognosis when it is expressed in both tumor tissue and serum in patients with gastric cancer [70]. It also intervenes in other MMPs function by up-regulating tumor-progression favorable ones such as MMP-1, MMP-7, and MMP-13 [71].

MMP-12 (matrix metalloelastase) is another metalloproteinase with dual role, more likely a protective one; it may be secreted by macrophages or by tumor cells, the biologic role being related with the type of secreting cell, thus it appears that macrophage-secreted MMP-12 has antitumor role, while tumor-secreted one has pro-tumor activity [72]. It was shown that MMP-12 knock-out mice grafted with B16 melanoma cells were more susceptible to develop TNF/IFN-induced inflammation than their wild-type counterparts [73] and its overexpression determines slower tumoral growth in experiments in mice [74]. As other elastases, it contributes to the releasing of angiogenic inhibitors from collagen fibers and angiostatin from plasminogen, thus exercising an anti-angiogenic activity [75–77]. Also, its anti-angiogenic effects may rely to uPAR cleavage [78] being a possible anti-tumoral therapeutic agent [79].

MMP-13 is involved in tumor progression most probable by increasing VEGF production in the tumor stroma. It is expressed both by tumor cells in invasive tumors and by tumor stroma. In experimental models of knocked-down MMP13 gene transgenic mice, it was showed that implants of melanoma cells (intradermal injection with B16F1 cell-line) develop smaller local tumors with less prominent vascularity after a longer period of time comparing with injected littermate controls (MMP-13+ mice); moreover, the incidence of metastases in mmp13–/– mice decreased dramatically in lung, liver, and brain being absent in the hearth as melanoma is known as one of the few tumors able to develop cardiac and spleen metastases; up to 40% of the control animal had cardiac metastases while none of the transgenic mice had such lesions [80, 81].

TIMPs (TIMP-1 to -4) are nodal biomolecules involved in epithelial-mesenchymal transition; since they are involved in several biological pathways their functions are more complex than simply modeling the extracellular matrix. Mostly, TIMPs regulates the activity of MMPs by binding to the catalytic sites of MMPs by their N-terminal domains forming a stoichiometric inhibitor complex; there is demonstrated selectivity of different types of TIMPs for specific type of MMPs. In case of MMP-2 and MMP-9, the C-terminal domain of TIMPs binds to the hemopexin-like domain of pro-MMP-2 and pro-MMP-9; replacement of C-terminal domain of TIMP-1 with either TIMP-2, TIMP-3 or TIMP-4 C-terminal domains improve TIMP-1 affinity for different MMPs (MMP14 and MMP19) and ADAMs (ADAM10 and ADAM17), inhibits TNF-α and HB-EGF shedding, inhibits cell migration in wound healing and eliminates the tumor growth effects of TIMP-1 [82–85].

TIMPs directly interact with cell adhesion molecules or directly intervene on cytoskeletal components, processes that alter both intercellular adhesion and cell growth. In addition, cellular proliferation is modulated by TIMPs direct interference with components of extracellular matrix [83, 86].

TIMPs are involved in angiogenesis, mostly with anti-angiogenic effects due to the modulation of MMPs activity. However, TIMP2 and TIMP-3 have supplemental effects in inhibiting angiogenesis. TIMP-2 inhibits proliferation and migration of endothelial cells and (either by interacting with $\alpha3\beta$ receptor or by inducing the RECK expression which subsequent inhibition of MMP-2, MMP-9, MT1-MMP, ADAM10). TIMP-3 blocks VEGF-A mitogenic actions and regulates VEGFR2 expression [23, 83, 86, 87].

Tumor growth effects of TIMPs are also related to their intervention in apoptosis, either pro- or anti-apoptotic molecules. TIMP-1 and TIMP-2 have antiapoptotic activity modulating PI3-kinase and JNK pathways (unrelated to TIMP-1 inhibition of MMP functions) while TIMP-3 stabilizes Fas and TNF-cell receptor 1 (proapoptotic effects) [23, 83, 86, 88].

2. MMPs and TIMPs role in response to treatment and resistance to therapeutic agents in melanoma

In melanoma treatment with acute BRAF inhibition, it was reported that active MMP-2, MT1-MMP, and MMP-9 are decreased, but it did not modulate TIMP-2 or RECK. Using cell models, it was shown that resistance to vemurafenib induces significant changes in the tumor microenvironment mainly by MMP-2 upregulation, but not upon TIMP expression, MMP up-regulation corresponding to an increase in cell invasiveness [89]. Another research group using experimental cell models by transfection of miR-21 and inducing over-expression in the melanoma cell lines WM1552c, WM793b, A375, and MEL 39 has shown that miR-21 decreases TIMP3 expression and enhances the invasiveness of melanoma cells. In an animal model, using 01B74 Athymic NCr-nu/nu mice, treatment with a miR-21 antagomir inhibited tumor growth and increased tumor expression of TIMP-3 [90].

3. MMPs and TIMPs expression in melanoma with regression

There are very few tumors that can present spontaneous regression up to the point of complete clinical and histopathologic vanishing. Melanoma is such a tumor, its disappearance reaching the point of impossibility of tumor cell identification even by immunohistochemical test; the indirect proof of previous existence of the tumor is represented by the presence of so-called tumor melanosis [91]. There different types of regression in melanoma are described: *complete regression* with total disappearance of tumor cells (immunohistochemistry fails to identified any neoplastic melanocyte, tumor being superseded by an area of fibrosis with hyperplastic blood vessels, and dense inflammatory infiltrate with numerous melanophages); *segmentary regression* (part of the tumor suffered complete regression); and *partial regression* (the regression is present but few tumor cells can be identified in the area, either morphologically or immunohistochemically) [92].

Regression is a phenomenon that occurs naturally relatively frequent in melanoma—up to 10–35% of cases; an even higher incidence was reported in thin melanomas—up to 60% of cases with a Breslow index of <0.75 mm [10, 92–94]. Despite these data, complete regression is reported in very few cases (mostly, as case reports and about 0.25% in large studies [95]); the real incidence of this phenomenon cannot be established since patients with completely regressed melanoma are not aware of the disease unless they develop distant metastasis. The biologic significance and prognosis of regression in melanoma is a matter of debate, various opinion being published [91, 96–105]. Mechanisms involved in occurring of regression in melanoma are yet to be deciphered; considering the importance of host response in this process, investigation of tumor microenvironment may offer some responses.

Study of MMPs and TIMPs expression in melanoma with regression was performed by our group by analyzing 93 melanomas (62 superficial spreading melanomas (SSM) and 31 nodular melanoma (NM)), 39 cases of SSM showing regression. Regression was present as both segmental and partial type, either pure form or combined (segmental regression (SR)—33.33%, partial regression (PR)—43.58%, and SR-PR in the same tumor—23.07%). Five MMPs and three TIMPs were analyzed (MMP-1, MMP-3, MMP-9, MMP-11, MMP-13, TIMP-1, TIMP-2, and TIMP-3) in both regressed and non-regressed areas of the tumors, the results being compared with those recorded in melanomas without regression (absence of regression—AR). A semi-quantitative score with four levels based on the level of staining intensity, namely "absent" (−), "mild positive" (+), "moderate positive" (++), and "intense positive" (+++) was used to assess the immunohistochemical expression of each marker in either tumor or stromal cells.

Two types of results were obtained: (a) differences in MMPs and TIMPs expression between non-regressed component of melanoma with regression (NRC) and melanoma without regression (AR) and (b) differences in MMPs and TIMPs expression between regressed component (RC) and NRC in melanoma with regression [106].

3.1. Differences in MMPs and TIMPs expression in tumor cells between NRC and AR

MMP-1 was intense positive (+++) in all AR melanomas; also, most of the NRC were intense positive (+++) for MMP-1, only 15.84% of them being moderately positive (++) (**Figure 1a–c**).

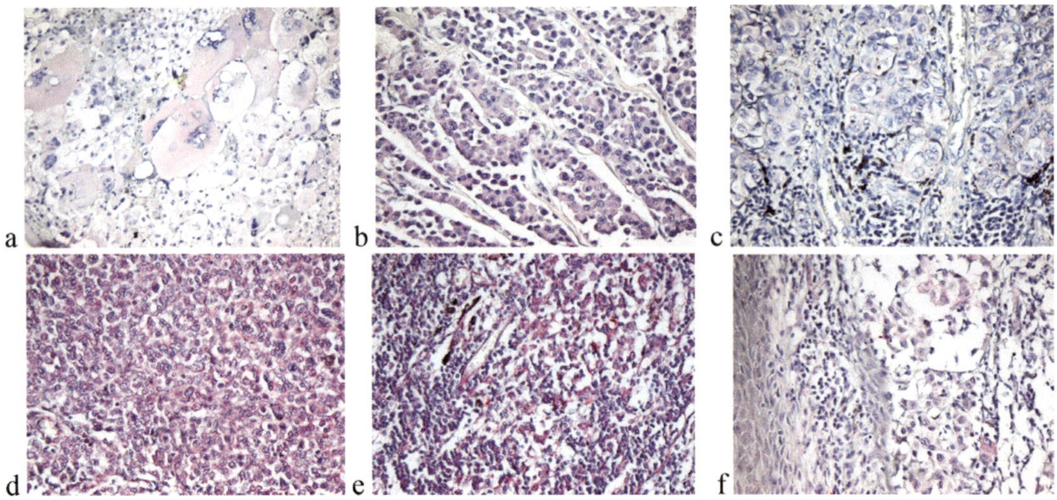

Figure 1. MMP-1 and MMP-11 (fast red detection): (a) melanoma without regression, faint diffuse positivity for MMP-1; monstrous tumor cells are more intense positive than main tumoral mass. MMP-1 × 200. (b) Melanoma with partial regression, faint diffuse positivity for MMP-1 in non-regressed component. MMP-1 × 200. (c) Melanoma with partial regression, faint diffuse positivity for MMP-1 in regressed component. MMP-1 × 400. (d) Melanoma with partial regression, faint diffuse positivity for MMP-11 in non-regressed component in both tumor and stromal cells. MMP-11 × 400. (e) Melanoma with partial regression, diffuse positivity for MMP-11 in regressed component in both tumor cells, endothelial cells and fibroblasts. MMP-11 × 400. (f) Melanoma with partial regression, faint positivity for MMP-11 in regressed component in both tumor cells. MMP-11 × 400.

Despite the small percentage of less positive cases for MMP-1 in melanomas with regression, this feature was statistically significant.

Similar findings as in case of MMP-1 were present for MMP-11 (**Figure 1d–f**): all AR cases were intense positive, while 74.35% of NRCs were intense positive, the rest (25.65%) being moderate positive; also, the tendency of a diminished expression of MMP-11 in NRC than in AR cases was statistically significant.

MMP-2 (**Figure 2a–c**), MMP-3 (**Figure 2d–f**), MMP-7 (**Figure 2g–i**), MMP-9 (**Figure 2j–l**), and MMP-13 (**Figure 2m–o**) showed similar features of diminished expression in NRC than in AR but the data were not statistically significant; data for MMP-13 expression had a level of statistical significance of 0.07.

No significant differences for TIMP-1 (**Figure 3a–c**), TIMP-2 (**Figure 3d–f**), and TIMP-3 (**Figure 3g–i**) expression were recorded between NRC and AR tumor cells.

Our study identified an overall diminished expression of MMP-1, MMP-3, MMP-9, MMP-11, and MMP-13 in NRC comparing to AR as control; since most of these biomolecules have pro-tumor activities, it is possible to speculate that they favor a less aggressive biologic behavior melanoma with regression.

There were differences when the specific type of regression was considered. Expression of MMP-1 in NRC of tumors with SR (either SR or combined SR-PR) was statistically significant diminished comparing with both AR cases or with NRC in PR cases. No such differences were

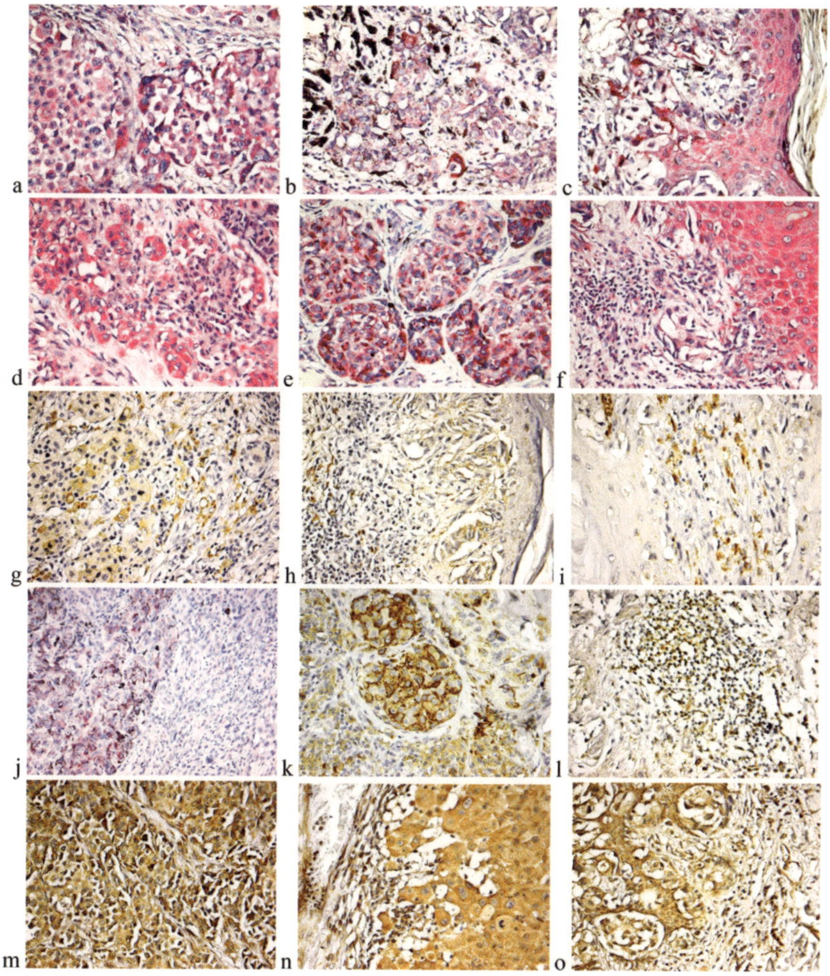

Figure 2. MMP-2, MMP-3, and MMP-7 (fast red detection), MMP-9 (fast red and DAB detection), MMP-13 (DAB detection): (a) melanoma without regression, diffuse positivity for MMP-2. MMP-2 × 400. (b) Melanoma with partial regression, diffuse positivity for MMP-2 in non-regressed component. MMP-2 × 400. (c) Melanoma with partial regression, diffuse positivity for MMP-2 in regressed component. MMP-2 × 400. (d) Melanoma without regression, diffuse positivity for MMP-3 in both tumor and stromal cells. MMP-3 × 400. (e) Melanoma with partial regression, diffuse positivity for MMP-3 in non-regressed component. MMP-3 × 400. (f) Melanoma with partial regression, diffuse positivity for MMP-3 in regressed component in both tumor and stromal cells. MMP-3 × 400. (g) Melanoma with partial regression, diffuse positivity for MMP-7 in non-regressed component in both tumor and stromal cells. MMP-7 × 400. (h) Melanoma with partial regression, diffuse positivity for MMP-7 in regressed component in both tumor and stromal cells. MMP-7 × 400. (i) Melanoma with segmental regression, intense positivity for MMP-7 in regressed component in stromal cells; no tumor cells are present. MMP-7 × 400. (j) Melanoma without regression, diffuse positivity for MMP-9; pigmented tumor cells are slightly more intense positive than nonpigmented ones. MMP-9 × 400 (fast red detection). (k) Melanoma with partial regression, diffuse positivity for MMP-9 in regressed component in tumor cells; few fibroblasts from area of regression are also positive; faint cytoplasmic positivity of plasma cells. MMP-9 × 400 (DAB detection). (l) Melanoma with segmental regression, positivity for MMP-9 in regressed component in inflammatory cells and fibroblasts; no tumor cells are present. MMP-9 × 400 (DAB detection). (m) Melanoma without regression, diffuse positivity for MMP-13; MMP-13 × 400. (n) Melanoma with partial regression, diffuse positivity for MMP-13 in non-regressed component in tumor cells, fibroblasts, endothelial and inflammatory cells. MMP-13 × 400. (o) Melanoma with partial regression, diffuse positivity for MMP-13 in regressed component in tumor cells; fibroblasts, endothelial and inflammatory cells from area of regression are also positive. MMP-13 × 400.

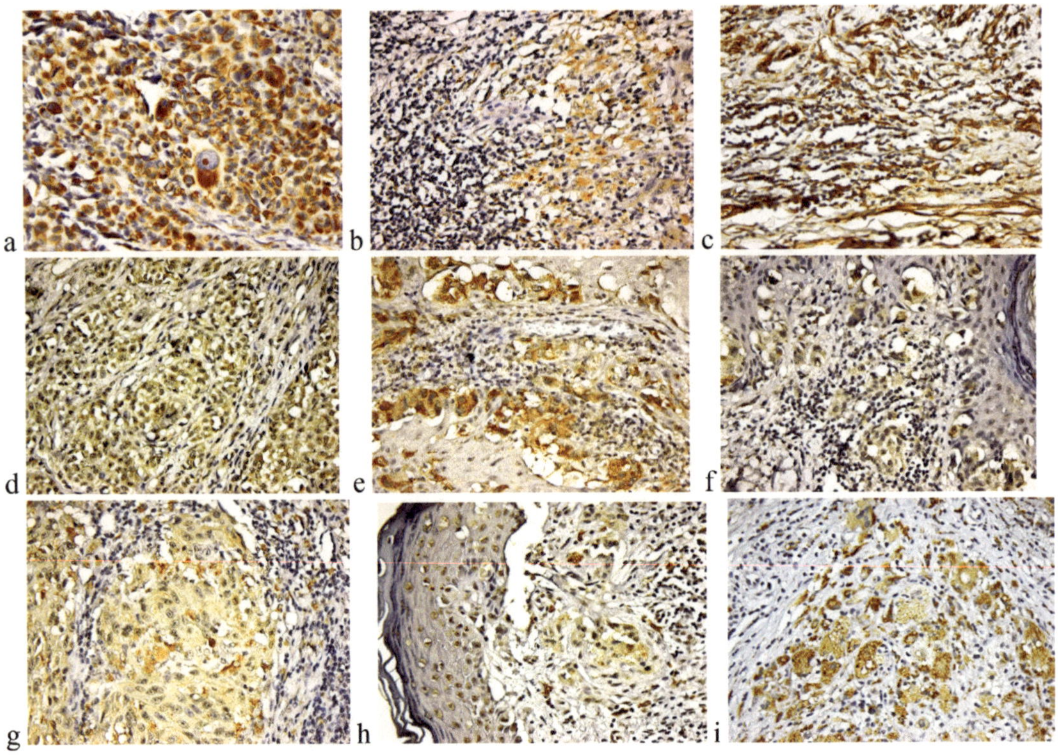

Figure 3. TIMP-1, TIMP-2, and TIMP-3 (DAB detection): (a) melanoma without regression, diffuse positivity for TIMP-1; TIMP-1 × 400. (b) Melanoma with partial regression, diffuse positivity for TIMP-1 in non-regressed component in tumor cells, few fibroblasts, few endothelial and few plasma cells. TIMP-1 × 400. (c) Melanoma with segmental regression, diffuse positivity for TIMP-1 in area of regression in fibroblasts, endothelial and inflammatory cells. TIMP-1 × 400. (d) Melanoma without regression, diffuse positivity for TIMP-2; TIMP-2 × 400. (e) Melanoma with partial regression, diffuse positivity for TIMP-2 in non-regressed component in tumor cells. TIMP-2 × 400. (f) Melanoma with partial regression, faint positivity for TIMP-2 in non-regressed component in tumor cells. TIMP-2 × 400. (g) Melanoma with partial regression, diffuse variable positivity for TIMP-3 in non-regressed component; TIMP-3 × 400. (h) Melanoma with partial regression, faint diffuse positivity for TIMP-3 in non-regressed component in tumor cells. TIMP-3 × 400. (i) Melanoma with partial regression, variable positivity for TIMP-3 in non-regressed component in tumor cells. TIMP-3 × 400.

noted for other MMPs (MMP2, MMP3, MMP11, and MMP13). Expression of TIMP-1 and/or TIMP-2 in NRC of tumors with PR was statistically significant increased comparing with either NRC of SR cases (TIMP-1 P = 0.011; TIMP-2 P = 0.009) or with NRC of SR-PR cases and AR (P = 0.002 and 0.037, respectively). There was no difference in TIMP-3 expression in NRC and/or AR cases according to the type of regression.

3.2. Differences in MMPs and TIMPs expression between RC and NRC in melanoma with regression

The differences in MMPs and TIMPs expression were evaluated in the same tumor, both in tumoral and stromal cells. In case of tumors with SR, the expression was evaluated in stromal cells (fibroblasts) present in regressed area. In the other cases (PR tumors, SR-PR tumors, and AR tumors), most of the cases showed similar expression of each marker in tumor cells versus stromal fibroblast for each tumor compartment.

In all the cases, there was either similar expression of MMPs in tumor cells in both areas (NRC and RC) or slightly overexpression in NRC comparing with RC. MMP-3 was the biomolecule with the most numerous cases of overexpression (76.93% had MMP-3 overexpression in NRC than in RC), followed by MMP-2 and MMP-11 (58.97% each), MMP-13 (48.71%), and MMP-1 (30.76%). Tumor stromal fibroblasts were also slightly more intense positive in NRC than in RC or showed similar expression in both components.

Considering the specific type of regression, MMP2 was over-expressed tumor fibroblasts in NRC than in RC in PR cases comparing with SR ones (P = 0.023). Also, differences occurred in case of MMP-13 expression—all SR-PR cases had MMP-13 overexpression in NRC versus RC comparing with PR and SR cases (P = 0.003, respectively, P = 0.0003). No significant differences occurred in case of MMP-1, MMP-3, and MMP-11 expression.

TIMPs expression had more variability in NRC versus RC component both in tumoral and stromal cells; there were cases with overexpression, similar expression or diminished expression for each type of TIMP investigated. However, most of the cases (66.66% for TIMP-1, 61.53% for TIMP-2, and 64.10% for TIMP-3) had TIMP overexpression in NRC versus RC.

The type of regression did not influence TIMP-1 and TIMP-2 expression in NRC and RC. In case of TIMP-3, all SR melanomas had TIMP-3 overexpression in stromal tumor fibroblasts in NRC when compared with those in RC component (P = 0.007).

4. Conclusions

Cancer biology is a complex phenomenon, several mechanisms concurring to tumor progression and metastasis. The role of the tumor microenvironment and its regulation by both tumor neoplastic cells and host response was lately established, the identification of several stromal-related biomarkers offering some explanations for different biology behavior of tumors with otherwise similar origin and classical histopathologic appearance.

MMPs and TIMPs are potent molecules involved in tumor development, progression, and metastasis with either pro- and anti-tumor activity; their correlation with regression in melanoma shows: (a) regressed and nonregressed components are in fact different tumor subclones and (b) in some cases of melanoma with regression (with a specific morphology), the biologic aggressiveness of the tumor and implicitly the overall prognosis may be more favorable than that of melanoma without regression, thus offering the possibility of a supplemental stratification of these patients beyond AJCC staging. More studies are needed to establish comprehensive pathways as a gate for identification of new biomarkers for either diagnostic or therapeutic purposes.

Acknowledgements

This paper is partially supported by Executive Agency for Higher Education, Research, Development and Innovation (UEFISCDI) under the contract number PN-III-P4-ID-PCE-2016-0641 (Project No. 183/2017).

Conflict of interest

The authors declare no conflict of interests.

Author details

Alexandra Bastian, Luciana Nichita and Sabina Zurac*

*Address all correspondence to: sabina_zurac@yahoo.com

Department of Pathology, University of Medicine and Pharmacy Carol Davila, Colentina University Hospital, Bucharest, Romania

References

[1] Siegel R, Naishadham D, Jemal A. Cancer statistics, 2012. CA: A Cancer Journal for Clinicians. 2012;**62**:10-29. DOI: 10.3322/caac.20138

[2] Balch CM, Gershenwald JE, Soong SJ, Thompson JF, Atkins MB, Byrd DR, Buzaid AC, Cochran AJ, Coit DG, Ding S, Eggermont AM, Flaherty KT, Gimotty PA, Kirkwood JM, McMasters KM, Mihm MC Jr, Morton DL, Ross MI, Sober AJ, Sondak VK. Final version of 2009 AJCC melanoma staging and classification. Journal of Clinical Oncology. 2009;**27**:6199-6206. DOI: 10.1200/JCO.2009.23.4799

[3] Pardoll DM. The blockade of immune checkpoints in cancer immunotherapy. Nature Reviews. Cancer. 2012;**12**:252-264. DOI: 10.1038/nrc3239

[4] Chapman PB, Hauschild A, Robert C, Haanen JB, Ascierto P, Larkin J, Dummer R, Garbe C, Testori A, Maio M, Hogg D, Lorigan P, Lebbe C, Jouary T, Schadendorf D, Ribas A, O'Day SJ, Sosman JA, Kirkwood JM, Eggermont AM, Dreno B, Nolop K, Li J, Nelson B, Hou J, Lee RJ, Flaherty KT, McArthur GA, BRIM-3 Study Group. Improved survival with vemurafenib in melanoma with BRAF V600E mutation. The New England Journal of Medicine. 2011;**364**:2507-2516. DOI: 10.1056/NEJMoa1103782

[5] Flaherty KT, Robert C, Hersey P, Nathan P, Garbe C, Milhem M, Demidov LV, Hassel JC, Rutkowski P, Mohr P, Dummer R, Trefzer U, Larkin JM, Utikal J, Dreno B, Nyakas M, Middleton MR, Becker JC, Casey M, Sherman LJ, Wu FS, Ouellet D, Martin AM, Patel K, Schadendorf D, METRIC Study Group. Improved survival with MEK inhibition in BRAF-mutated melanoma. The New England Journal of Medicine. 2012;**367**:107-114. DOI: 10.1056/NEJMoa1203421

[6] Schadendorf D, Amonkar MM, Stroyakovskiy D, Levchenko E, Gogas H, de Braud F, Grob JJ, Bondarenko I, Garbe C, Lebbe C, Larkin J, Chiarion-Sileni V, Millward M, Arance A, Mandalà M, Flaherty KT, Nathan P, Ribas A, Robert C, Casey M, DeMarini DJ, Irani JG, Aktan G, Long GV. Health-related quality of life impact in a randomised phase

III study of the combination of dabrafenib and trametinib versus dabrafenib monotherapy in patients with BRAF V600 metastatic melanoma. European Journal of Cancer. 2015;**51**:833-840. DOI: 10.1016/j.ejca.2015.03.004

[7] Long GV, Stroyakovskiy D, Gogas H, Levchenko E, de Braud F, Larkin J, Garbe C, Jouary T, Hauschild A, Grob JJ, Chiarion-Sileni V, Lebbe C, Mandalà M, Millward M, Arance A, Bondarenko I, Haanen JB, Hansson J, Utikal J, Ferraresi V, Kovalenko N, Mohr P, Probachai V, Schadendorf D, Nathan P, Robert C, Ribas A, DeMarini DJ, Irani JG, Swann S, Legos JJ, Jin F, Mookerjee B, Flaherty K. Dabrafenib and trametinib versus dabrafenib and placebo for Val600 BRAF-mutant melanoma: A multicentre, double-blind, phase 3 randomised controlled trial. Lancet. 2015;**386**:444-451. DOI: 10.1016/S0140-6736(15)60898-4

[8] Long GV, Stroyakovskiy D, Gogas H, Levchenko E, de Braud F, Larkin J, Garbe C, Jouary T, Hauschild A, Grob JJ, Chiarion-Sileni V, Lebbe C, Mandalà M, Millward M, Arance A, Bondarenko I, Haanen JB, Hansson J, Utikal J, Ferraresi V, Kovalenko N, Mohr P, Probachai V, Schadendorf D, Nathan P, Robert C, Ribas A, DeMarini DJ, Irani JG, Swann S, Legos JJ, Jin F, Mookerjee B, Flaherty K. Combined BRAF and MEK inhibition versus BRAF inhibition alone in melanoma. The New England Journal of Medicine. 2014;**371**:1877-1888. DOI: 10.1056/NEJMoa1406037

[9] Chen ST, Geller AC, Tsao H. Update on the epidemiology of melanoma. Current Dermatology Reports. 2013;**2**:24-34. DOI: 10.1007/s13671-012-0035-5

[10] Gimotty PA, Botbyl J, Soong SJ, Guerry DJ. Population-based validation of the AJCC melanoma staging system. Clinical Oncology. 2005;**23**:8065-8075. DOI: 10.1200/JCO.2005.02.4976

[11] McKinnon JG, Yu XQ, McCarthy WH, Thompson JF. Prognosis for patients with thin cutaneous melanoma: Long-term survival data from New South Wales central cancer registry and the Sydney Melanoma Unit. Cancer. 2003;**98**:1223-1231. DOI: 10.1002/cncr.11624

[12] Balch CM, Soong SJ, Gershenwald JE, Thompson JF, Reintgen DS, Cascinelli N, Urist M, McMasters KM, Ross MI, Kirkwood JM, Atkins MB, Thompson JA, Coit DG, Byrd D, Desmond R, Zhang Y, Liu PY, Lyman GH, Morabito A. Prognostic factors analysis of 17,600 melanoma patients: Validation of the American Joint Committee on cancer melanoma staging system. Journal of Clinical Oncology. 2001;**19**:3622-3634. DOI: 10.1200/JCO.2001.19.16.3622

[13] Gimotty PA, Elder DE, Fraker DL, Botbyl J, Sellers K, Elenitsas R, Ming ME, Schuchter L, Spitz FR, Czerniecki BJ, Guerry D. Identification of high-risk patients among those diagnosed with thin cutaneous melanomas. Journal of Clinical Oncology. 2007;**25**:1129-1134. DOI: 10.1200/JCO.2006.08.1463

[14] Checinska A, Soengas MS. The gluttonous side of malignant melanoma: Basic and clinical implications of macroautophagy. Pigment Cell & Melanoma Research. 2011;**24**:1116-1132. DOI: 10.1111/j.1755-148X.2011.00927.x

[15] Murphy-Ullrich JE. The de-adhesion activity of matricellular proteins: Is intermediate cell adhesion an adaptive state? The Journal of Clinical Investigation. 2001;**107**:785-790

[16] Hsu MY, Shih DT, Meier FE, Van Belle P, Hsu JY, Elder DE, Buck CA, Herlyn M. Adenoviral gene transfer of β3 integrin subunit induces conversion from radial to vertical growth phase in primary human melanoma. The American Journal of Pathology. 1998;**153**:1435-1442

[17] Straume O, Akslen LA. Importance of vascular phenotype by basic fibroblast growth factor, and influence of the angiogenic factors basic fibroblast growth factor/fibroblast growth factor receptor-1 and ephrin-A1/EphA2 on melanoma progression. The American Journal of Pathology. 2002;**160**:1009-1019

[18] Hanahan D, Weinberg RA. Hallmarks of cancer: The next generation. Cell. 2011;**144**: 646-674

[19] Egeblad M, Nakasone ES, Werb Z. Tumors as organs: Complex tissues that interface with the entire organism. Developmental Cell. 2010;**18**:884-901

[20] Pietras K, Ostman A. Hallmarks of cancer: Interactions with the tumor stroma. Experimental Cell Research. 2010;**316**:1324-1331

[21] Kessenbrock K, Plaks V, Werb Z. Matrix metalloproteinases: Regulators of the tumor microenvironment. Cell. 2010;**141**:52-67

[22] Caley MP, Martins VLC, O'Toole EA. Metalloproteinases and wound healing. Advances in Wound Care (New Rochelle). 2015;**4**:225-234

[23] Visse R, Nagase H. Matrix metalloproteinases and tissue inhibitors of metalloproteinases: Structure, function, and biochemistry. Circulation Research. 2003;**92**:827-839. DOI: 10.1161/01.RES.0000070112.80711.3D

[24] Slootweg PJ, Zurac S. Prognostic and predictive value of epithelial to mesenchymal transition-associated markers in oral squamous cell carcinoma. Current Proteomics. 2013;**10**:218-227. DOI: 10.2174/1570164611310030004

[25] Milner JM, Cawston TE. Matrix metalloproteinase knockout studies and the potential use of matrix metalloproteinase inhibitors in the rheumatic diseases. Current Drug Targets. Inflammation and Allergy. 2005;**4**:363-375

[26] Sternlicht MD, Werb Z. How matrix metalloproteinases regulate cell behavior. Annual Review of Cell and Developmental Biology. 2001;**17**:463-516

[27] Mannello F, Medda V. Nuclear localization of matrix metalloproteinases. Progress in Histochemistry and Cytochemistry. 2012;**47**:27-58

[28] Gialeli C, Theocharis AD, Karamanos NK. Roles of matrix metalloproteinases in cancer progression and their pharmacological targeting. The FEBS Journal. 2011;**278**:16-27

[29] Nagase H, Woessner JF. Matrix metalloproteinases. The Journal of Biological Chemistry. 1999;**274**:21491-21494

[30] Kalluri R, Weinberg RA. The basics of epithelial-mesenchymal transition. The Journal of Clinical Investigation. 2009;**119**:1420-1428

[31] Airola K, Karonen T, Vaalamo M, Lehti K, Lohi J, Kariniemi AL, Keski-Oja J, Saarialho-Kere UK. Expression of collagenases-1 and -3 and their inhibitors TIMP-1 and -3 correlates with the level of invasion in malignant melanomas. British Journal of Cancer. 1999;**80**:733-743. DOI: 10.1038/sj.bjc.6690417

[32] Blackburn JS, Rhodes CH, Coon CI, Brinckerhoff CERNA. Interference inhibition of matrix metalloproteinase-1 prevents melanoma metastasis by reducing tumor collagenase activity and angiogenesis. Cancer Research. 2007;**67**:10849-10858. DOI: 10.1158/008-5472.CAN-07-1791

[33] Blackburn JS, Liu I, Coon CI, Brinckerhoff CE. A matrix metalloproteinase-1/protease activated receptor-1 signaling axis promotes melanoma invasion and metastasis. Oncogene. 2009;**28**:4237-4248. DOI: 10.1038/onc.2009.272

[34] Boire A, Covic L, Agarwal A, Jacques S, Sherifi S, Kuliopulos A. PAR1 is a matrix metalloprotease-1 receptor that promotes invasion and tumorigenesis of breast cancer cells. Cell. 2005;**120**:303-313. DOI: 10.1016/j.cell.2004.12.018

[35] Wandel E, Grasshoff A, Mittag M, Haustein UF, Saalbach A. Fibroblastssurrounding melanoma express elevated levels of matrix metalloproteinase-1 (MMP-1) and intercellular adhesion molecule-1 (ICAM-1) *in vitro*. Experimental Dermatology. 2000;**9**:34-41

[36] Goerge T, Barg A, Schnaeker EM, Poppelmann B, Shpacovitch V, Rattenholl A, Maaser C, Luger TA, Steinhoff M, Schneider SW. Tumor-derived matrix metalloproteinase-1 targets endothelial proteinase-activated receptor 1 promoting endothelial cell activation. Cancer Research. 2006;**66**:7766-7774

[37] Hoyhtya M, Hujanen E, Turpeenniemi-Hujanen T, Thorgeirsson U, Liotta LA, Tryggvason K. Modulation of type-IV collagenase activity and invasive behavior of metastatic human melanoma (A2058) cells in vitro by monoclonal antibodies to type IV collagenase. International Journal of Cancer. 1990;**46**:282-286

[38] Kurschat P, Zigrino P, Nischt R, Breitkopf K, Steurer P, Klein CE, Krieg T, Mauch C. Tissue inhibitor of matrix metalloproteinase-2 regulates matrix metalloproteinase-2 activation by modulation of membrane-type 1 matrix metalloproteinase activity in high and low invasive melanoma cell lines. The Journal of Biological Chemistry. 1999;**274**:21056-21062

[39] Kurschat P, Wickenhauser C, Groth W, Krieg T, Mauch C. Identification of activated matrix metalloproteinase-2 (MMP-2) as the main gelatinolyticenzyme in malignant melanoma by in situ zymography. The Journal of Pathology. 2002;**197**:179-187. DOI: 10.1002/path.1080

[40] Hofmann UB, Eggert AA, Blass K, Bröcker EB, Becker JC. Stromal cells as the major source for matrix metalloproteinase-2 in cutaneous melanoma. Archives of Dermatological Research. 2005;**297**:154-160. DOI: 10.1007/s00403-005-0588-2

[41] Ntayi C, Hornebeck W, Bernard P. Influence of cultured dermal fibroblasts on human melanoma cell proliferation, matrix metalloproteinase-2 (MMP-2) expression and invasion in vitro. Archives of Dermatological Research. 2003;**295**:236-241. DOI: 10.1007/s00403-003-0429-0

[42] Jiao Y, Feng X, Zhan Y, Wang R, Zheng S, Liu W, Zeng X. Matrix metalloproteinase-2 promotes alpha vbeta3 integrin-mediated adhesion and migration of human melanoma cells by cleaving fibronectin. PLoS One. 2012;**7**:e41591. DOI: 10.1371/journal.pone.0041591

[43] Rotte A, Martinka M, Li G. MMP2 expression is a prognostic marker for primary melanoma patients. Cellular Oncology (Dordrecht). 2012;**35**:207-216. DOI: 10.1007/s13402-012-0080-x

[44] Vaisanen A, Tuominen H, Kallioinen M, Turpeenniemi-Hujanen T. Matrix metalloproteinase-2 (72 kD type IV collagenase) expression occurs in the early stage of human melanocytic tumour progression and may have prognostic value. The Journal of Pathology. 1996;**180**:283-289

[45] Turpeenniemi-Hujanen T. Gelatinases (MMP-2 and -9) and their natural inhibitors as prognostic indicators in solid cancers. Biochimie. 2005;**87**:287-297

[46] Hofmann UB, Westphal JR, Zendman AJ, Becker JC, Ruiter DJ, van Muijen GN. Expression and activation of matrix metalloproteinase-2 (MMP-2) and its co-localization with membrane-type 1 matrix metalloproteinase (MT1-MMP) correlate with melanoma progression. The Journal of Pathology. 2000;**191**:245-256

[47] Krengel S, Alexander M, Brinckmann J, Tronnier M. MMP-2, TIMP-2 and MT1-MMP are differentially expressed in lesional skin of melanocytic nevi and their expression is modulated by UVB-light. Journal of Cutaneous Pathology. 2002;**29**:390-396

[48] Su F, Bradley WD, Wang Q, Yang H, Xu L, Higgins B, Kolinsky K, Packman K, Kim MJ, Trunzer K, Lee RJ, Schostack K, Carter J, Albert T, Germer S, Rosinski J, Martin M, Simcox ME, Lestini B, Heimbrook D, Bollag G. Resistance to selective BRAF inhibition can be mediated by modest upstream pathway activation. Cancer Research. 2012;**72**:969-978. DOI: 10.1158/0008-5472.CAN-11-1875

[49] Benbow U, Schoenermark MP, Mitchell TI, Rutter JL, Shimokawa K, Nagase H, Brinckerhoff CEA. Novel host/tumor cell interaction activates matrixmetalloproteinase 1 and mediates invasion through type I collagen. The Journal of Biological Chemistry. 1999;**274**:25371-25378

[50] Nikkola J, Vihinen P, Vlaykova T, Hahka-Kemppinen M, Kähäri VM, Pyrhönen S. High expression levels of collagenase-1 and stromelysin-1 correlate with shorter disease-free survival in human metastatic melanoma. International Journal of Cancer. 2002;**97**:432-438

[51] Witty JP, Lempka T, Coffey RJ Jr, Matrisian LM. Decreased tumor formation in 7,12-dimethylbenzanthracene-treated stromelysin-1 transgenic mice is associated with alterations in mammary epithelial cell apoptosis. Cancer Research. 1995;**55**:1401-1406

[52] Kivisaari AK, Kallajoki M, Ala-aho R, McGrath JA, Bauer JW, Königová R, Medvecz M, Beckert W, Grénman R, Kähäri VM. Matrix metalloproteinase-7 activates heparin-binding epidermal growth factor-like growth factor in cutaneous squamous cell carcinoma. The British Journal of Dermatology. 2010;**163**:726-735. DOI: 10.1111/j.1365-2133.2010.09924.x

[53] Pines G, Köstler WJ, Yarden Y. Oncogenic mutant forms of EGFR: Lessons in signal transduction and targets for cancer therapy. FEBS Letters. 2010;**584**:2699-2706. DOI: 10.1016/j.febslet.2010.04.019

[54] Felli N, Felicetti F, Lustri AM, Errico MC, Bottero L, Cannistraci A, De Feo A, Petrini M, Pedini F, Biffoni M, Alvino E, Negrini M, Ferracin M, Mattia G, Carè A. miR-126 & -126* restored expressions play a tumor suppressor role by directly regulating ADAM9 and MMP7 in melanoma. PLoS One. 2013;**8**:e56824. DOI: 10.1371/journal.pone.0056824

[55] Kawasaki K, Kawakami T, Watabe H, Itoh F, Mizoguchi M, Soma Y. Expression of matrilysin (matrix metalloproteinase-7) in primary cutaneous and metastatic melanoma. The British Journal of Dermatology. 2007;**156**:613-619. DOI: 10.1111/j.1365-2133.2006.07678.x

[56] Montel V, Kleeman J, Agarwal D, Spinella D, Kawai K, Tarin D. Altered metastatic behavior of human breast cancer cells after experimental manipulation of matrix metalloproteinase 8 gene expression. Cancer Research. 2004;**64**:1687-1694

[57] Decock J, Long JR, Laxton RC, Shu XO, Hodgkinson C, Hendrickx W, Pearce EG, Gao YT, Pereira AC, Paridaens R, Zheng W, Ye S. Association of matrix metalloproteinase-8 gene variation with breast cancer prognosis. Cancer Research. 2007;**67**:10214-10221

[58] Gutiérrez-Fernández A, Fueyo A, Folgueras AR, Garabaya C, Pennington CJ, Pilgrim S, Edwards DR, Holliday DL, Jones JL, Span PN, Sweep FC, Puente XS, López-Otín C. Matrix metalloproteinase-8 functions as a metastasis suppressor through modulation of tumor cell adhesion and invasion. Cancer Research. 2008;**68**:2755-2763. DOI: 10.1158/0008-5472.CAN-07-5154

[59] Lopez-Otin C, Palavalli LH, Samuels Y. Protective roles of matrix metallo-proteinases: From mouse models to human cancer. Cell Cycle. 2009;**8**:3657-3662

[60] Palavalli LH, Prickett TD, Wunderlich JR, Wei X, Burrell AS, Porter-Gill P, Davis S, Wang C, Cronin JC, Agrawal NS, Lin JC, Westbroek W, Hoogstraten-Miller S, Molinolo AA, Fetsch P, Filie AC, O'Connell MP, Banister CE, Howard JD, Buckhaults P, Weeraratna AT, Brody LC, Rosenberg SA, Samuels Y. Analysis of the matrix metalloproteinase family reveals that MMP8 is often mutated in melanoma. Nature Genetics. 2009;**41**:518-520. DOI: 10.1038/ng.340

[61] Balbín M, Fueyo A, Tester AM, Pendás AM, Pitiot AS, Astudillo A, Overall CM, Shapiro SD, López-Otín C. Loss of collagenase-2 confers increased skin tumor susceptibility to male mice. Nature Genetics. 2003;**5**:252-257

[62] Coussens LM, Tinkle CL, Hanahan D, Werb Z. MMP 9 supplied by bone marrow-derived cells contributes to skin carcinogenesis. Cell. 2000;**103**:481-490

[63] Takeha S, Fujiyama Y, Bamba T, Sorsa T, Nagura H, Ohtani H. Stromal expression of MMP 9 and urokinase receptor is inversely associated with liver metastasis and with infiltrating growth in human colorectal cancer: A novel approach from immune/inflammatory aspect. Japanese Journal of Cancer Research. 1997;**88**:72-81

[64] Scorilas A, Karameris A, Arnogiannaki N, Ardavanis A, Bassilopoulos P, Trangas T, Talieri M. Overexpression of matrix metalloproteinase 9 in human breast cancer: A potential favourable indicator in node-negative patients. British Journal of Cancer. 2001; **4**:1488-1496

[65] Hamano Y, Zeisberg M, Sugimoto H, Lively JC, Maeshima Y, Yang C, Hynes RO, Werb Z, Sudhakar A, Kalluri R. Physiological levels of tumstatin, a fragment of collagen IV $\alpha3$ chain, are generated by MMP 9 proteolysis and suppress angiogenesis via $\alpha V\beta3$ integrin. Cancer Cell. 2003;**3**:589-601

[66] Lopez-Otin C, Matrisian LM. Emerging roles of proteases in tumor suppression. Nature Reviews. Cancer. 2007;**7**:800-808

[67] Bodey B, Bodey B Jr, Siegel SE, Kaiser HE. Matrix metalloproteinase expression in malignant melanomas: Tumor-extracellular matrix interactions in invasion and metastasis. In Vivo. 2001;**15**:57-64

[68] Ramos MC, Steinbrenner H, Stuhlmann D, Sies H, Brenneisen P. Induction of MMP-10 and MMP-1 in a squamous cell carcinoma cell line by ultraviolet radiation. Biological Chemistry. 2004;**385**:75-86. DOI: 10.1515/BC.2004.010

[69] Boyd S, Virolainen S, Pärssinen J, Skoog T, van Hogerlinden M, Latonen L, Kyllönen L, Toftgard R, Saarialho-Kere U. MMP-10 (Stromelysin-2) and MMP-21 in human and murine squamous cell cancer. Experimental Dermatology. 2009;**18**:1044-1052. DOI: 10.1111/j.1600-0625.2009.00901.x

[70] Aung PP, Oue N, Mitani Y, Nakayama H, Yoshida K, Noguchi T, Bosserhoff AK, Yasui W. Systematic search for gastric cancer-specific genes based on SAGE data: Melanoma inhibitory activity and matrix metalloproteinase-10 are novel prognostic factors in patients with gastric cancer. Oncogene. 2006;**25**:2546-2557. DOI: 10.1038/sj.onc.1209279

[71] Pittayapruek P, Meephansan J, Prapapan O, Komine M, Ohtsuki M. Role of matrix metalloproteinases in photoaging and photocarcinogenesis. International Journal of Molecular Sciences. 2016;**17**:E868. DOI: 10.3390/ijms17060868

[72] Houghton AM, Grisolano JL, Baumann ML, Kobayashi DK, Hautamaki RD, Nehring LC, Cornelius LA, Shapiro SD. Macrophage elastase (matrix metalloproteinase-12) suppresses growth of lung metastases. Cancer Research. 2006;**66**:6149-6155. DOI: 10.1158/0008-5472. CAN-04-0297

[73] Van Roy M, Van Lint P, Van Laere I, Wielockx B, Wilson C, López-Otin C, Shapiro S, Libert C. Involvement of specific matrix metalloproteinases during tumor necrosis factor/IFN gamma-based cancer therapy in mice. Molecular Cancer Therapeutics. 2007;**6**:2563-2571. DOI: 10.1158/1535-7163.MCT-07-0016

[74] Martin MD, Matrisian LM. The other side of MMPs: Protective roles in tumor progression. Cancer Metastasis Reviews. 2007;**26**:717-724. DOI: 10.1007/s10555-007-9089-4

[75] Sund M, Xie L, Kalluri R. The contribution of vascular basement membranes and extracellular matrix to mechanics of tumor angiogenesis. APMIS. 2004;**112**:450-462. DOI: 10.1111/ j.1600-0463.2004.t01-1-apm11207-0806.x

[76] Ribatti D. Endogenous inhibitors of angiogenesis: A historical review. Leukemia Reearch. 2009;**33**:638-644. DOI: 10.1016/j.leukres.2008.11.019

[77] Xu Z, Shi H, Li Q, Mei Q, Bao J, Shen Y, Mouse XJ. Macrophage metalloelastase generates angiostatin from plasminogen and suppresses tumor angiogenesis in murine colon cancer. Oncology Reports. 2008;**20**:81-88

[78] Andolfo A, English WR, Resnati M, Murphy G, Blasi F, Sidenius N. Metalloproteases cleave the urokinase-type plasminogen activator receptor in the D1-D2 linker region and expose epitopes not present in the intact soluble receptor. Thrombosis and Haemostasis. 2002;**88**:298-306

[79] Laurenzana A, Biagioni A, D'Alessio S, Bianchini F, Chillà A, Margheri F, Luciani C, Mazzanti B, Pimpinelli N, Torre E, Danese S, Calorini L, Del Rosso M, Fibbi G. Melanoma cell therapy: Endothelial progenitor cells as shuttle of the MMP12 uPAR-degrading enzyme. Oncotarget. 2014;**5**:3711-3727. DOI: 10.18632/oncotarget.1987

[80] Lederle W, Hartenstein B, Meides A, Kunzelmann H, Werb Z, Angel P, Mueller MM. MMP13 as a stromal mediator in controlling persistent angiogenesis in skin carcinoma. Carcinogenesis. 2010;**31**:1175-1184. DOI: 10.1093/carcin/bgp248

[81] Zigrino P, Kuhn I, Bäuerle T, Zamek J, Fox JW, Neumann S, Licht A, Schorpp-Kistner M, Angel P, Mauch C. Stromal expression of MMP-13 is required for melanoma invasion and metastasis. The Journal of Investigative Dermatology. 2009;**129**:2686-2693. DOI: 10.1038/jid.2009.130

[82] Duan JX, Rapti M, Tsigkou A, Lee MH. Expanding the activity of tissue inhibitors of metalloproteinase (TIMP)-1 against surface-anchored metalloproteinases by the replacement of its C-terminal domain: Implications for anti-cancer effects. PLoS One. 2015;**10**:e01363842015. DOI: 10.1371/journal.pone.0136384

[83] Zurac S, Neagu M, Constantin C, Cioplea M, Nedelcu R, Bastian A, Popp C, Nichita L, Andrei R, Tebeica T, Tanase C, Chitu V, Caruntu C, Ghita M, Popescu C, Boda D, Mastalier B, Maru N, Daha C, Andreescu B, Marinescu I, Rebosapca A, Staniceanu F, Negroiu G, Ion DA, Nikitovic D, Tzanakakis GN, Spandidos DA, Tsatsakis AM. Variations in the expression of TIMP1, TIMP2 and TIMP3 in cutaneous melanoma with regression and their possible function as prognostic predictors. Oncology Letters. 2016;**11**:3354-3360. DOI: 10.3892/ol.2016.4391

[84] Brew K, Dinakarpandian D, Nagase H. Tissue inhibitors of metalloproteinases: Evolution, structure and function. Biochimica et Biophysica Acta. 2000;**1477**:267-283

[85] Bourboulia D, Stetler-Stevenson WG. Matrix metalloproteinases (MMPs) and tissue inhibitors of metalloproteinases (TIMPs): Positive and negative regulators in tumor cell adhesion. Seminars in Cancer Biology. 2010;**20**:161-168

[86] Baker AH, Edwards DR, Murphy G. Metalloproteinase inhibitors: Biological actions and therapeutic opportunities. Journal of Cell Science. 2002;**115**:3719-3727. DOI: 10.1242/jcs.00063

[87] Paul-Samojedny M, Pudełko A, Suchanek-Raif R, Kowalczyk M, Fila-Daniłow A, Borkowska P, Kowalski J. Knockdown of the AKT3 (PKBγ), PI3KCA, and VEGFR2 genes by RNA interference suppresses glioblastoma multiforme T98G cells invasiveness *in vitro*. Tumour Biology. 2015;**36**:3263-3277. DOI: 10.1007/s13277-014-2955-0

[88] Guo LJ, Luo XH, Xie H, Zhou HD, Yuan LQ, Wang M, Liao EY. Tissue inhibitor of matrix metalloproteinase-1 suppresses apoptosis of mouse bone marrow stromal cell line MBA-1. Calcified Tissue International. 2006;**78**:285-292. DOI: 10.1007/s00223-005-0092-x

[89] Sandri S, Faião-Flores F, Tiago M, Pennacchi PC, Massaro RR, Alves-Fernandes DK, Berardinelli GN, Evangelista AF, de Lima Vazquez V, Reis RM, Maria-Engler SS. Vemurafenib resistance increases melanoma invasiveness and modulates the tumor microenvironment by MMP-2 upregulation. Pharmacological Research. 2016;**111**:523-533. DOI: 10.1016/j.phrs.2016.07.017

[90] Martin del Campo SE, Latchana N, Levine KM, Grignol VP, Fairchild ET, Jaime-Ramirez AC, Dao TV, Karpa VI, Carson M, Ganju A, Chan AN, Carson WE 3rd. MiR-21 enhances melanoma invasiveness via inhibition of tissue inhibitor of metalloproteinases 3 expression: *In vivo* effects of MiR-21 inhibitor. PLoS One. 2015;**10**:e0115919. DOI: 10.1371/journal.pone.0115919

[91] Alquier-Bouffard A, Franck F, Joubert-Zakeyh J, Barthélémy I, Mansard S, Ughetto S, Aublet-Cuvelier B, Déchelotte PJ, Mondié JM, Souteyrand P, D'incan M. Regression in primary cutaneous melanoma is not predictive for sentinel lymph node micrometastasis. Annales de Dermatologie et de Vénéréologie. 2007;**134**:521-525

[92] Zurac S, Negroiu G, Petrescu S, Andrei R, Tebeica T, Popp C, Mustată R, Neagu M, Constantin C, Solovan C, et al. Spectrum of morphologic alterations of regression in cutaneous melanoma-potential for improving disease prognosis. Romanian Journal of Internal Medicine. 2012;**50**:145-153

[93] McGovern VJ, Shaw HM, Milton GW. Prognosis in patients with thin malignant melanoma: Influence of regression. Histopathology. 1983;**7**:673-680

[94] Abramova L, Slingluff CL Jr, Patterson JW. Problems in the interpretation of apparent "radial growth phase" malignant melanomas that metastasize. Journal of Cutaneous Pathology. 2002;**29**:407-414

[95] Balch CM, Buzaid AC, Soong SJ, Atkins MB, Cascinelli N, Coit DG, Fleming ID, Gershenwald JE, Houghton A Jr, Kirkwood JM, McMasters KM, Mihm MF, Morton DL, Reintgen DS, Ross MI, Sober A, Thompson JA, Thompson JF. Final version of the American joint committee on cancer staging system for cutaneous melanoma. Journal of Clinical Oncology. 2001;**19**:3635-3648. DOI: 10.1200/JCO.2001.19.16.3635

[96] Trau H, Kopf AW, Rigel DS, Levine J, Rogers G, Levenstein M, Bart RS, Mintzis MM, Friedman RJ. Regression in malignant melanoma. Journal of the American Academy of Dermatology. 1983;**8**:363-368

[97] Kaur C, Thomas RJ, Desai N, Green MA, Lovell D, Powell BW, Cook MG. The correlation of regression in primary melanoma with sentinel lymph node status. Journal of Clinical Pathology. 2008;**61**:297-300

[98] Shaw HM, Rivers JK, McCarthy SW, McCarthy WH. Cutaneous melanomas exhibiting unusual biologic behavior. World Journal of Surgery. 1992;**16**:196-202

[99] Guitart J, Lowe L, Piepkorn M, Prieto VG, Rabkin MS, Ronan SG, Shea CR, Tron VA, White W, Barnhill RL. Histological characteristics of metastasizing thin melanomas: A case-control study of 43 cases. Archives of Dermatology. 2002;**138**:603-608

[100] Blessing K, McLaren KM. Histological regression in primary cutaneous melanoma: Recognition, prevalence and significance. Histopathology. 1992;**20**:315-322

[101] Paladugu RR, Yonemoto RH. Biologic behavior of thin malignant melanomas with regressive changes. Archives of Surgery. 1983;**118**:41-44

[102] Oláh J, Gyulai R, Korom I, Varga E, Dobozy A. Tumour regression predicts higher risk of sentinel node involvement in thin cutaneous melanomas. The British Journal of Dermatology. 2003;**149**:662-663

[103] Socrier Y, Lauwers-Cances V, Lamant L, Garrido I, Lauwers F, Lopez R, Rochaix P, Chevreau C, Payoux P, Viraben R, Paul C, Meyer N. Histological regression in primary melanoma: Not a predictor of sentinel lymph node metastasis in a cohort of 397 patients. The British Journal of Dermatology. 2010;**162**:830-834. DOI: 10.1111/j.1365-2133.2009.09606.x.

[104] Fontaine D, Parkhill W, Greer W, Walsh N. Partial regression of primary cutaneous melanoma: Is there an association with sub-clinical sentinel lymph node metastasis? The American Journal of Dermatopathology. 2003;**25**:371-376

[105] Liszkay G, Orosz Z, Péley G, Csuka O, Plótár V, Sinkovics I, Bánfalvi T, Fejõs Z, Gilde K, Kásler M. Relationship between sentinel lymph node status and regression of primary malignant melanoma. Melanoma Research. 2005;**15**:509-513

[106] Andrei R, Zurac S, Socoliuc C, Staniceanu F. Variation in expression of metalloproteinases in cutaneous melanoma with regression, possible indicator of tumor heterogeneity. DermatoVenerol (Buc). 2015;**60**:133-145

Section 5

Role of Matrix Metalloproteinases in Wound Healing

Chapter 8

Biological Activity and Implications of the Metalloproteinases in Diabetic Foot Ulcers

Claudia Castruita-De la Rosa, Idalia Garza-Veloz,
Edith Cardenas-Vargas,
Rodrigo Castañeda-Miranda, Luis O. Solis-Sanchez,
Jose M. Ortiz-Rodriguez, Hector R. Vega-Carrillo,
Maria R. Martinez-Blanco, Virginia Flores-Morales,
Gloria P. Hernandez-Delgadillo,
Jose I. Badillo-Almaráz and
Margarita L. Martinez-Fierro

Additional information is available at the end of the chapter

http://dx.doi.org/10.5772/intechopen.71725

Abstract

Inadequate metabolic control predisposes diabetic patient to a series of complications on account of diabetes mellitus (DM). Among the most common complications of DM is neuropathy, which causes microvascular damage by hyperglycemia in the lower extremities which arrives characterized by a delayed closing. The global prevalence of diabetic neuropathy (DN) was 66% of people with diabetes in 2015, representing the principal cause of total or partial lower extremities amputation, with 22.6% of the patients with DN. Matrix metalloproteinases (MMPs) are involved in healing. The function that these mainly play is the degradation during inflammation that has as consequence the elimination of the extracellular matrix (ECM), the disintegration of the capillary membrane to give way to angiogenesis and cellular migration for the remodeling of damaged tissue. The imbalance in MMPs may increase the chronicity of a wound, what leads to chronic foot ulcers and amputation. This chapter focuses on the role of MMPs in diabetic wound healing.

Keywords: MMPs, wounds, diabetic foot

1. Introduction

Diabetes mellitus (DM) is a set of metabolic disorders, characterized by the presence of persistently elevated blood glucose levels caused by a deficiency of insulin production or insulin resistance [1]. Chronic hyperglycemia is related to the appearance of microvascular complications, knowing as diabetic neuropathy (DN) that compromises the metabolism, inducing the formation of end products of advanced glycosylation and reactive oxygen species and reduction of the elimination of free radicals and endothelial dysfunction with neuronal damage. DN is a set of alterations that affect both the sensory and motor fibers as the autonomous system. Hyperglycemia is invariably associated with alterations in nerve conduction and the feet are highly susceptible to initiate phases of hypoesthesia. Vasomotor control is lost and blood flow to the extremity (vasodilation of the veins of the dorsum of the foot) is increased, but this flow is channeled into the skin and arteriovenous fistulas in the bone, which can cause hypoperfusion in other tissues. When normal capillary reflexes are lost, capillary hypertension of dependence and a decreased vasodilatory response to heat occur. Increased blood flow causes demineralization and bone osteopenia [2]. The diabetic foot ulcer (DFU) is the most common complication of lower limb DM. It is also the most disabling late complication of the disease. The World Health Organization (WHO) defines it as "a syndrome in which complications of a diverse etiology: neuropathic, vascular and infectious stemming from DM and predisposing to the suffering and development of ulcers."

There are more than 347 million people with DM in the world, of which 66% had DN in 2015, representing one of the principal causes of 22.6% total or partial lower extremities amputation [3]. DFU is considered as the major epidemic disease in the last decade; its etiological factors are DN and arterial disease. Neuropathy alone in 46%, ischemia in 12% being the most frequent neuroischemia (60%) and no risk factor identified in 12%. About 15% of diabetic patients will have ulcers in the lower extremities, half of these patients who have a single ulcer will subsequently develop another ulcer, and one third of these ulcers will cause limb amputation [4]. The worldwide DFU prevalence ranges from 1.3% to 4.8%. The current medical treatments for these chronic wounds continue to be somewhat opposed according to the country and the international guides that govern [5]. Part of the affections that these ulcers generate is in the extracellular matrix (MEC), where the matrix metalloproteases (MMP) are able to degrade all the components of MEC. The MMPs are indispensable for the healing process; among its functions is to eliminate the provisional extracellular matrix and facilitate migration to the wound center; they also participate in the remodeling of granulation tissue in the control of angiogenesis and the release of some growth factors [6, 7]. Different types of MMP expression patterns are present in a wound; it has been shown that immunity processes, such as cell migration, participate in the process of re-epithelialization and in the formation of scars [8]. Accordingly, the correct expression and regulation of MMPs are related with the healing process and therefore with a successful process of cicatrization.

2. Contents

2.1. Matrix metalloproteinases (MMPs)

The MMPs belong to a family of zinc-containing endopeptidases are calcium dependent, capable of degrading and remodeling the proteins that form the ECM and carry out different biological and physiological functions; they are regulated by hormones, growth factors and cytokines [9]. Based on their specificity for the components of the MEC, MMPs are divided into collagenases, gelatinases, stromelysins and matrilysins. A numeric system has been adapted for the MMPs grouping them according to their structure and give place to eight different structural classes of MMPs. This system groups in five different groups those MMPs that are secreted, and in three groups to those MMPs according to their type of membrane, acquiring as MTP-MMP identification [10]. The first group of the minimal domain MMPs contains an amino-terminal signal sequence (Pre) that directs them to the endoplasmic reticulum, a propeptide (Pro) with a thiol group (SH) that interacts with the zinc and maintains them as inactive zymogens and a catalyst with a zinc binding site (Zn). The second group in addition to a minimal domain also contains a hemopexin-like domain that is connected to the catalytic domain by a hinge (H), which mediates interactions with the tissue inhibitors of the MMPs. The first and last of the four replicates in the hemopexin-like domain are linked by a disulfide bond (S-S). The third group of gelatinase-binding MMPs contains inserts resembling fibronectin (Fi) type II collagen-binding repeats. The fourth group of MMPs is furin (Fu) secreted and contains a recognition motif for serine and Fu type intracellular proteinases between their polypeptide and catalytic domains that allow intracellular activation by these proteinases. Within the fifth group is the vitronectin-like insert (Vn). The number group is included in membrane MMP (MT-MMP); these are conformed by a carboxy-terminal single chain (TM) transmembrane domain, a very short cytoplasmic domain (Cy). The seventh group has MMPs that are anchored in glycosylphosphatidylinositol (GPI), and within group eight MMP-23 is included, is membrane bound, has an N-terminal signal (SA) that targets the cell membrane, and therefore in a type II transmembrane MMP, and is characterized by a single domain of cysteine (CA) and immunoglobulin (Ig) [11]. This is shown in **Figure 1** [11].

In mammalian, MMPs are inhibited by four metalloproteinase tissue inhibitors (TIMPs), which are endogenous regulators of MMP family proteins, whose function is to determine the influence of ECM, cell adhesion molecules, cytokines, chemokines and growth factors. TIMPs are formed by an amino-terminal (N-terminal) domain, which is the inhibition domain that binds to the active site of MMPs, and a subdomain C. The capacity of these TIMPs to inhibit MMPs is due to the interaction in the N-terminal domain that binds within the cleft of the active site of the target MMP. The C-domain has two parallel β strands that are connected by an α-helix to two anti-parallel β strands. This structure provides the ability of TIMPs to interact with the hemopexin domain of some MMP [12].

There are four TIMP family members: TIMP-1, -2, -3 and TIMP-4; each of its N and C domains, in their final position, possess six cysteine residues, which constitute three disulfide domains. The N-terminal region is assembled into the catalytic domain of MMPs where the action of MMP will be inhibited; in the case of the C region, it binds to the proformas of a domain called hemopexin C—in its terminal position for the case of the MMP-2,9 and thus binds to a pro-enzyme complex inhibitor. For TIMP-2, this binds specifically to the surface of the cell with TIM-1MMP and pro MMP-2, this to carry out the activation of the

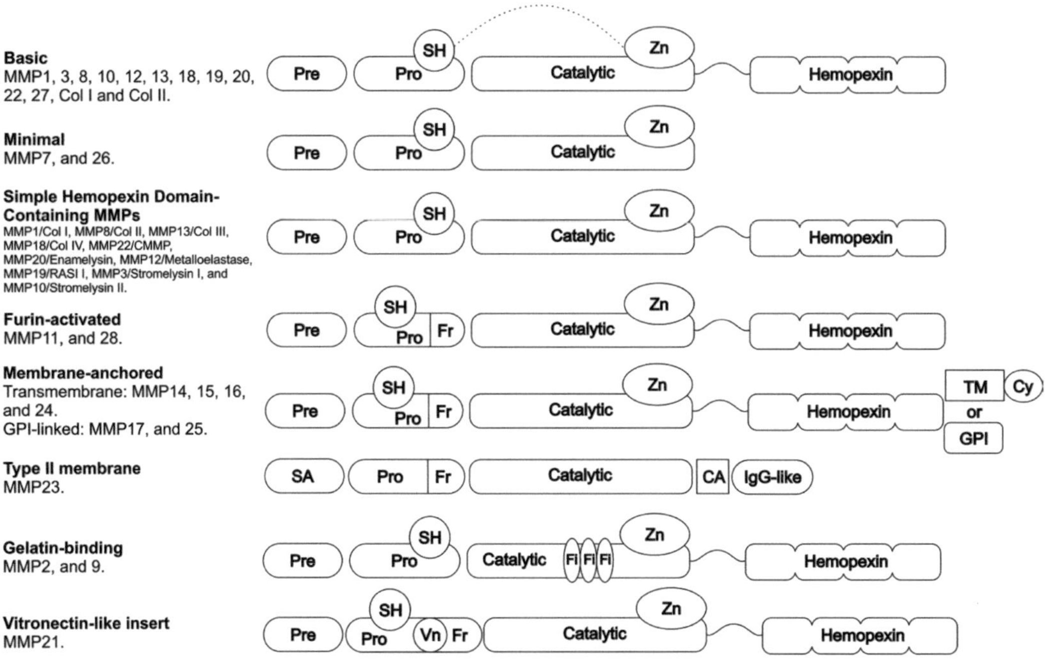

Figure 1. Domain structure of MMP groups. All human MMPs show the signal peptide, the pro-domain and the catalytic domain. Pre = pre-domain (contains the signal peptide) and Pro = pro-domain, which contains cysteine sequence that complexes Zn^{2+} in the zymogen form. The catalytic region contains the center domain. Fr = furin cleavage, Fi = fibronectin repeat, Vn = vitronectin-like insert, Cy = cytosolic, CA = cysteine array, Hemopexin = hemopexin domain, IgG-like = Ig-like domain, TM = transmembrane domain and GPI = glycosylphosphatidylinositol anchor. The hemopexin domain is linked to the catalytic center by a hinge region.

pro-MMP-2 in a simple way [13]; as consequently, TIMP-2 is an inhibitor that also functions as an activator of MMPs. The four TIMPs can inactivate the already active MMPs, but they will not do so with the same effectiveness. MMP-1,3,7 and 9 are inhibited by TIMP-1, in the case of TIMP-2 inactive to MMP-2. TIMP-3 is inactivating MMP-2,9 but similarly to the ADAM group, finally TIMP-4 inactivates MT1-MMP and MMP-2. Therefore, in regard to the function of TIMPs is the regular proteolysis activity and in those functions related to the activities of the MMPs [14]. The role of TIMP1 is expressed in mammalian tissues, specifically in reproductive organs; TIMP2 is constitutively expressed in most tissues, but not inducible by growth factors and TIMP3 is expressed in tissues as a matrix protein. TIMP4 is expressed relatively in heart, ovary, pancreas, colon and testes [12], where they observed the specific expression constitutively or inducible, which is regulated at transcriptional level by cytokines and growth factors [15]. It has been proposed to have a relevant role in processes including cell proliferation, adhesion and migration and/or apoptosis by cutting bioactive molecules that modulate these processes [16]. MMPs modulate biological processes during pathophysiological events, such as skeletal formation, angiogenesis, cell migration, inflammation, wound healing, coagulation, pulmonary and cardiovascular diseases, arthritis and cancer. They have been identified in human degrading components of ECM, cellular receptors and cytokines [17].

2.2. Regulation of MMP activity

In normal physiological conditions, the activity of MMPs is accurately regulated at four levels. (1) *Transcription*. The transcription of MMPs is induced by various exogenous signals, including cytokines, growth factors, chemical agents, physical stress and oncogenic cellular transformation, and also by cell-matrix and cell-cell interactions. The genes that control MMPs respond to extracellular signals (MMP-1, MMP-13, MMP-3, MMP-10, MMP-7, MMP-12 and MMP-9), which possess an AP-1 (activator of the protein-1) in the promoter proximal to the position −70 of the site of initiation of the transcription [18, 19]. The promoter regions of the MMP-2 and MMP-11 genes do not contain an AP-1 element [20]. The promoter region of membrane type 1-matrix metalloproteinase (MT1-MMP) gene lacks of AP-1 element, but it contains Sp-1 binding site which is essential for MT1-MMP transcription [21]. (2) *Activation of precursor zymogens*. For the regulation of MMPs by a zymogen, a biochemical change is required to turn an inactive enzyme into an active enzyme. Propeptides that maintain MMPs in their zymogen form (proMMP) can be activated by proteinases or *in vitro* by chemical agents. Proteolysis is initiated in the exposed region between the first and second propellants of a propeptide, following the specificity of the region followed by the sequence in each MMP. After the initiation of proteolysis, a part of the propeptide is separated; this unbalances the rest of the propeptide, including the cysteine-zinc interaction and allows the intermolecular process that is carried out by activated MMP mediators [22]. Plasmin is generated from the plasminogen by means of the tissue plasminogen activator, which is bound to fibrin and to a urokinase activator attached to the cellular receptor. Plasminogen being the plasminogen enhancer of the urokinase is bound to the membrane, generating pro-MMP activation such as proMMP-1, 3,7,9,10,13 and ECM movement [23]. (3) *Interaction with specific components of ECM*. The location, action and specificity of the MMPs generate an association with the components of the NDE. One of the functions of MMPs may be the destruction of ECM in tissues. The ECM has the function of storing active biological molecules as they are growth factors [11]. For example, the degradation of type I collagen by collagenase is associated with osteoclast activation and keratinocyte migration during re-epithelialization [24]. (4) *Inhibition by TIMPs*. TIMPs are specific inhibitors that bind MMPs in a 1:1 stoichiometry and their expression is regulated during development and tissue remodeling. Under pathological conditions associated with unbalanced MMP activities, changes of TIMP levels are considered to be important because they directly affect the level of MMP activity. TIMPs are specific inhibitors that bind MMPs in a 1:1 stoichiometry; their expression is regulated during development and tissue remodeling. Under pathological conditions associated with unbalanced MMP activities, changes of TIMP levels are considered to be important because they directly affect the level of MMP activity. The proteolytic activity of MMPs is inhibited specifically by TIMPs and by nonspecific proteinase inhibitors, such as a 1-proteinase inhibitor and α2-macroglobulin. TIMPs are the major endogenous regulators of MMP activity in tissue, which are expressed by different cell types, including fibroblasts, keratinocytes, endothelial cells and osteoblasts. As inhibitors of MMPs, TIMPs maintain the balance between the ECM deposition and degradation in physiological and pathological processes [22].

2.3. Wound repair

Wound repair is a physiological event, in which tissue injury results in a repair process that finally leads to restoration of structure and function of the tissue [25]. During wound healing, the degradation of the components of the ECM by MMP is necessary to remove and rearrange the provisional matrices and allow cell migration [26]; thus, basal keratinocytes are the predominant source of MMP. Cutaneous wound repair can be divided into three overlapping phases: (i) formation of fibrin clot followed by inflammation, (ii) re-epithelialization and granulation tissue formation and iii) matrix formation and remodeling [27].

2.3.1. Formation of fibrin clot followed by inflammation

The first step for wound repair is a fibrin clot formed through platelet aggregation and blood coagulation. The coagulation cascades are initiated by coagulation factors of the injured skin, this by means of the extrinsic system. The thrombocytes are activated to generate aggregation by means of exposed collagen, this being controlled by the intrinsic system. Following this, the injured vessels continue with a vasoconstriction of 5 or 10 minutes, being triggered by platelets; this to reduce blood loss and begin to fill the void of tissue that was generated by the wound through a compound clot cytokines and growth factors [28]. Vasoconstriction generates clots, followed by vasodilation, where thrombocytes invade the wound matrix on a provisional basis [27]. The formed clot contains fibrin molecules, fibronectin, vitronectin and thrombospondin, forming the provisional matrix as a scaffold structure for the migration of leukocytes, keratinocytes, fibroblasts and endothelial cells [29]. Platelets influence leukocyte infiltration; this is mediated by the synthesis of factors for chemotaxis. Platelets and leukocytes release cytokines and growth factors for activation of the inflammation process. The interleukins IL-1α, β, IL-6 and TNF-α are involved, such as FGF-b, IGF, TGF-β are involved in the process of collagen synthesis, factors such as FGF-B, VEGF subunit A, HIF-1 and TGF-β are involved for angiogenesis and for the EGF, FGF-b, IGF, TGF-α [30]. See **Figure 2**.

2.3.2. Proliferation and re-epithelialization

In the proliferation phase, the main focus of the healing process is to cover the wound surface, to form granulation tissue and to restore the vascular network. After to tissue injury, platelets are recruited to the injury site to stop the bleeding. Platelets also release platelet-derived growth factor (PDGF) that initiates the migration of neutrophils and macrophages, in addition to causing the synthesis of growth factors and related cytokines in wound healing [31]. This factor is also involved in the stimulation of collagenase and in fibroblastic cell of human skin, with MMP-8 being more frequent in tissue damage [18]. The MMP-1,2,3,9 are synthesized by platelets; the function of MMP-1,2 aid in the balance of platelet adhesion and the conglomeration thereof [27]. In the inflammatory process, cells such as neutrophils are involved in the wound to protect infections and generate the synthesis and stimulation of MMP-8, being necessary for wound debridement and division of damaged type I collagen; the MMP-9 also participates by separating the collagen types that also participate (IV, V and X) [5].

Through the control of regulatory cytokines such as IFN-γ and TGF-β, the synthesis of collagen, fibronectin and other basic substances necessary for the healing of fibroblast wounds

http://dx.doi.org/10.5772/intechopen.71725

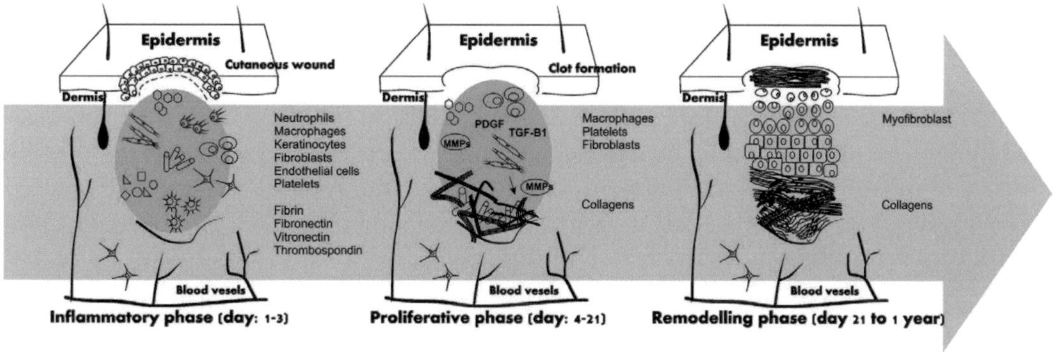

Figure 2. Wound repair phases. The wound repair phases involve: 1. Formation of the clot. The fibrin clot is being formed through platelet aggregation, coagulation cascades, fibrin molecules, fibronectin, vitronectin and thrombospondin to form a temporary scaffold for the initiation of leukocyte, keratinocyte, fibroblast and endothelial cell migration. 2. Proliferative phase. The platelets initiate the synthesis of MMPs 1, 2, 3, 9; MMP-1 and MMP-2 generate a balance in the adhesion of platelets and secrete PDGF initiating the migration of neutrophils, macrophages and growth factors. This generates the stimulation of different types of collagen, which are separated with the help of MMP-9. This stimulation of collagen is given by fibroblastic cells to begin the healing process and cover the surface of the wound. 3. Remodeling phase. In the remodeling of granulation tissue, there is an increase in the synthesis of collagen generating a decrease in fibroblasts. The keratinocytes initiate their migration to the clot through the granulation tissue to initiate tissue repair.

represents the basis for the new connective tissue matrix. Therefore, the migration of local fibroblasts along the fibrin network and the initiation of re-epithelialization from the wound edges, neovascularization and angiogenesis are activated by capillary sprouting [27]. This process is activated by signaling pathways of epithelial and non-epithelial cells at the wound edges, which release a myriad of different cytokines and growth factors such as EGF, KGF, IGF-1 and NGF [30].

In the process of re-epithelialization participate, the laminin is a component basal of the epithelium and plays roles in cell adhesion, migration, proliferation, differentiation and angiogenesis. There are 15 isoforms of laminin, of which laminin-5 is specific to epithelial cells. Laminin-5 has been shown to promote keratinocyte migration and induction of MMP-9; cell motility depends on MMP-9 activity, indicating that MMP-9 plays a role in re-epithelialization [32]. It is known that MMP-2 and MMP-14 cleave laminin-5 [33, 34] generating a fragment that binds to the epidermal growth factor receptor (EGF), which stimulates cell migration. The released FGF-2 from macrophages binds to heparan sulfate, which induces the growth of fibroblasts and endothelial cells [30]. Platelets and macrophages release vascular endothelial growth factor (VEGF), stimulating proliferation and migration of endothelial cells, as well as keratinocyte migration where are involved the MMP-1, MMP-2, MMP-9, and MMP-13 this plays a critical role in wound healing [35, 36].

2.3.3. Matrix formation and remodeling

Remodeling is the last phase of wound healing and occurs from day 21 to 1 year after injury. The collagen synthesis increases throughout the wound, whereas fibroblast proliferation decreases successively, adjusting a balance between synthesis and degradation of ECM [37]. This shows a signal. It gives a retraction and reorganization of filaments in the intracellular tone towards cell migration, where the keratinocytes migrate into the fibrin clot by infiltrating the upper layers of the granulation tissue [38]. The onset of granulation tissue repair is stopped by apoptosis, since in an old wound it is characterized by the absence of vascular structures within it and by having only ECM and having absence of cells [39]. In the case of maturation of a wound, type III collagen is displaced by collagen type I [40]. In the early stages of the remodeling phase, the provisional wound matrix contains predominantly fibrin and fibronectin, which are subsequently replaced by proteoglycan and collagen type I and III molecules, increases the tensile strength of the scar matrix. Fibroblasts are stimulated to transform into myofibroblasts that contract the wound matrix. At the end of the remodeling stage, the high density of blood vessels and myofibroblasts decrease with apoptosis. At the end of the process, the wound is completely closed [41, 42].

2.4. Proteolysis in wound repair

The proteolytic degradation of ECM is necessary in many stages of wound repair, such as interim matrix degradation, angiogenesis, keratinocyte migration and remodeling of granulation tissue ECM [43]. MMP-28 and MMP-19 are found in keratinocytes in the basal strata and suprabasals of healthy skin in an *in vivo* model [44]; in addition, MMP-19 is also found in hair follicles, endothelial cells and in veins and arteries [45]. In some wounds, the basal membrane is destroyed; this lesion temporarily retains MMP-1 expression in migratory cells that are expressed in the dermis, such as keratinocytes, with absence of a basement membrane [46]. The synthesis of MMP-1 is paramount for the initiation of re-epithelialization, so keratinocytes bind with type I collagen. Native type I collagen is known to generate MMP-1 synthesis in cells in vitro, contrary to basement membrane proteins such as fibronectin or collagen type III that do not generate this synthesis of MMP-1 [47].

MMP-1 is important in the process of migration of keratinocytes into native type I collagen and its synthesis, which is being generated by $\alpha 2\beta 1$ integrin [24]. In humans, the $\alpha 2\beta 1$-MMP-1 complex is to function as a motor stimulating migration of keratinocytes on type I collagen during re-epithelialization. Subsequent to the initiation of re-epithelialization, a new basement membrane is generated; here, the expression of MMP-1 in epidermis is arrested by cellular junctions with basement membrane proteins [47]. The role of MMP-1 in the wound healing process has been demonstrated in murine models, where there has been a delay in total wound [48].

Collagenase-3 (MMP-13) has been found in human skin, and it is related to the role of wound healing in the dermis. MMP-13 is synthesized by fibroblasts in those human cutaneous fetal wounds [49]. MMP-1 and MMP-13 can also regulate the survival of fibroblasts during dermal wound healing (affecting fibroblasts), which is mediated by matrix shrinkage and matrix rigidity [50]. MMP-8 is expressed by neutrophils, being stored in the cellular granules and being secreted to the outside by the activation thereof. In excessive skin wounds, the MMP-8

http://dx.doi.org/10.5772/intechopen.71725

is overexpressed [52]. Some experimental models in MMP-13-deficient knockout mice demonstrate that there is a MMP-13 compensation for MMP-8, demonstrating a delay in wound healing due to impaired re-epithelialization, low level of infiltration of neutrophils and a persistent inflammatory syndrome [51, 52].

The stromelysins, MMP-3 and MMP-10, are expressed by epidermal cells during wound repair in human and mouse wounds. MMP-3 is expressed by the basal proliferating keratinocytes behind migrating cells, whereas MMP-10 migration occurs by keratinocyte leaf [53]. MMP-3 can destroy substrates of the ECM, basement membrane proteins, in addition to increasing the activity and availability of cytokines and growth factors such as FGF-b and HB-EGF [22]. This poses a role for MMP-3 in the organization of the new basement membrane and in the involvement of cell migration and proliferation. The remodeling of the basement membrane after re-epithelialization, and degradation of the fibrin containing the provisional matrix, MMP-9 may be involved in the final adjustment of the epidermal tissue after wound healing by remodeling the cell [54].

MMP-2, 9, MT1-MMP and MMP-19 are synthesized in endothelial cells [55, 56]. Within these, MMP-2 and 9 have key participation in physiological aspects such as those tumorigenic and angiogenic processes [57]. These MMPs are responsible for degrading components of the vascular basement membrane, which is essential for the generation of new blood vessels. These MMPs physiologically participate in the activation of growth factors and cytokines related to angiogenesis [30]. MT1-MMP when involved in the generation of blood vessels is related to fibrinolytic and collagenolytic activity to generate invasion of these new vessels by crossing fibrin barriers in the stroma of damaged tissue [58]. MMP-19 is involved in the proliferation of epithelial tissue, endothelial cells, fibroblast cells and microvascular cells in macrophages [59]. See **Figure 2**.

2.5. MMPs in chronic wounds

Chronic wounds are defined as wounds where healing is delayed due to one or more factors. Depending on the etiology, a wound is considered to be chronic if it is still present after 4–6 weeks [60]. Such wounds may from the outset show chronic features, for example leg ulcers, pressure ulcers (PUs), DFUs and amputation stumps, or may initially be acute in nature (such as surgical wounds and traumatic wounds) and become chronic after several weeks of stagnation due to the patient's general condition or inappropriate care; they may last for several months or years.

The MMPs implicated in the wound healing process are listed in **Table 1**.

Chronic wounds present higher levels of protease activity than acute wounds. This has been demonstrated through comparative trials analyzing MMP levels in different populations. Chronic wounds, including venous leg ulcers (VLUs) [40, 61, 62], DFUs [63, 64], PUs [65] dehiscent surgical wounds and acute wounds that have become chronic, were found to have elevated MMP activity.

Type of MMPs	Subgroup of MMPs	Metalloprotease
Soluble gelatinases	Gelatinases	MMP-2: Gelatinase-A
		MMP-9: Gelatinase-B
Archetypal MMPs	Collagenases	MMP-1: Collagenase-1, interstitial collagenase
		MMP-8: Collagenase-2, neutrophil collagenase
		MMP-13: Collagenase-3
	Metalloelastase	MMP-12
	Stromelysins	MMP-3: Stromelysin-1
		MMP-10: Stromelysin-2
		MMP-11: Stromelysin-3
Matrilysins	Matrilysins	MMP-7: Matrilysin
		MMP-26: Matrilysin-2

MMP, matrix metalloproteinase.

Table 1. The main MMPs is involved into the wound healing process.

There is evidence that associates DM to changes in the foot structure, including abnormalities in fiber structure and organization, increased tendon thickness, volume and a tendency of impairing biomechanical properties [66]. Interestingly, these alterations may represent features of the ECM, which is in a constant state of dynamic equilibrium between synthesis and degradation. Besides the relevance of MMPs in the ECM and their role in the pathophysiology, data linking these proteases to the development and progression of diabetic disorders are still scarce. It has been found strong expression of MMP-13 and MMP-3 in diabetic foot ulcer both in diabetic and healthy, whereas MMP-13 expression was upregulated and MMP-3 expression decreased in the diabetic ulcer healing model. Moreover, upregulation of MMP-9 and MMP-13 and increased enzymatic activity of MMP-9 in a model *in vitro* treated with high glucose concentration is found [67].

As a result, it was obtained that at high glucose concentrations collagen degradation is induced by overproduction of MMPs, which leads to a vulnerable tissue [68]. Adding the MMPs also to the process of generation of diabetic fibrosis, this being a pathology differentiated by the excess of MMPs in the ECM generating changes in the same. This is a result of an imbalance between MMPs and TIMPs activity tissue such as hyperglycemia, dyslipidemia and hypertension [69], but increased production of collagen and other ECM components may also be involved. In fact, recruitment of inflammatory cells have been connected to dysregulation of homeostasis fibroblasts followed by secretion of ECM proteins, which results in an increased turnover and remodeling of the ECM. Moreover, MMPs are able to increase release of TGF-β1, which results in fibroblast cell proliferation and collagen I

http://dx.doi.org/10.5772/intechopen.71725

degradation [70]. Therefore, the relationship between MMP/TIMP may be associated with the development of diabetic ulcer as a consequence of poor regulation of ECM [69]. It is known that during DM there is no efficient wound healing; this being a consequence of the complications that occur in the metabolism and being a greater production of gelatinases in diabetes as a result of a period of inflammation [71]. MMPs are present in the degradation of the ECM, but also participate in the recovery of the trauma and promoting the renewal of the tissue. Likewise, the relationship with collagen is involved in the pathogenesis of the diabetic ulcer, implying poor tissue regeneration through a decrease in MMP-3 [71].

2.6. MMP levels in diabetic wound healing

Persistent hyperglycemia in the blood of diabetic patients induces the majority of the micro- and macrovascular complications associated with DM [20] and increases MMP activity directly or indirectly through oxidative stress or advanced glycation end products (AGEs) [72, 73]. An increased activity of MMPs may initiate the development of diabetic peripheral arterial disease. Hyperglycemia affects the regulation of MMP/TIMP and increases the activities of MMP-1, MMP-2 and MMP-9 in vascular cells, stimulating the degradation of the ECM and causing an imbalance in diabetes [74]. An increase in expression of MMP-2 and MMP-9 as well as protein expression of TIMP-1 may be a resulting factor in impaired wound healing and might provide an explanation for human arterial vasculature in type 2 DM [73].

The significantly higher levels of MMP in patients with metabolic syndrome as compared with normal individuals indicate that such patients may have high tendencies of developing other physiological problems [75]. The process of wound healing necessitates ECM degradation to be controlled; thus, an imbalance between ECM formation and the degradation process could lead to the development of chronic ulcers or fibrosis [76]. Cellular and biochemical imbalances, tissue damage, or other disease conditions may present varied effects in the healing process. This also upsets the proteases, cytokines, and growth factors leading to an absence or delay of wound closure preventing successful skin repair [72].

Enzyme activity affected by hyperglycemia disrupts the expression of MMPs in diabetes, and this generates an increased proteolytic environment provoked by an alteration in MMPs and TIMPs that affects patients with diabetic ulcers [77]. In healthy tissues, the levels of MMPs and TIMP are low; however, their synthesis and the activation of these are stimulated at the time of the remodeling of a tissue. In healthy skin, only the constitutive MMP-3, 7, 19, 28 and TIMP-1 expression has been documented [78]. Increased levels of MMP-1, MMP-8 and MMP-9 have been associated with a slow epithelial regeneration to heal wounds, with relatively low TIMP levels. MMP-9 degrades fibronectin into fragments, which further activates MMP, cell migration and proliferation. This provokes white blood cell infiltration, tissue damage and continuous inflammation. MMP-1, MMP-8 and MMP-9 are highly expressed in venous wounds in the absence of TIMPs [79, 80]. In addition, overexpression of MMP-9 and MMP-2 has been found in serum of patients with metabolic syndrome. The altered expression of MMPs may provoke pathogenesis in several tissues [75, 81]; the altered gene expression in MMP-9 is a cause of non-healing diabetic ulcers, being augmented in diabetic patients and not found in healthy patients [52], and MMP-1, MMP-2, MMP-8 and MMP-9 were highly expressed in normal and chronic diabetic wounds with a decrease in TIMP-2 [63]. This could be due to high proteolytic surroundings promoting poor healing in diabetes. Similarly, there was an overexpression of MMP-1 and MMP-9, as well as TIMP-1, in keratinocytes derived from foot ulcers in diabetic type 1 patients, supporting the theory on the upregulation of MMPs and TIMPs in diabetic foot ulcers [78]. Increased expression of MMP-9, TNF-α and other growth factors in DFUs has been found and concluded that they could be linked with slow-to-heal ulcers in diabetics and therefore a target for new therapeutic management [71].

Ascertained that MMPs and TIMPs are elevated in chronic wounds; however, they may also play a role in determining the level of chronicity. Yadav et al. [75] elucidated that chronicity is associated with an increase mainly in MMP-9 and MMP-8 and elastase activity that may eventually alter collagen synthesis and the release of growth factor and cytokines into the site of injury [82].

2.7. MMPs, prediction and healing in DFUs

MMPs are associated with wound healing. Investigating its expression in chronic wounds helps to generate a better evaluation in the prognostic aspect for diabetic foot ulcers; in this way, this knowledge assists in the investigation of aspects for the inhibition of these. DFUs often fail to heal, and the mechanism is not well explained. Normal wound healing is a complex process involving a highly orchestrated cascade of events that include hemostasis, inflammation, proliferation, angiogenesis and remodeling. In each of these events, the ECM interacts with growth factors and cells. Delayed healing is characterized by an increase in MMPs and a decrease in the levels of TIMPs and growth factors (specifically transforming growth factor TGF-β). MMPs and TIMPs are synthesized by cells associated with wound healing, where their concentrations vary according to the stage of healing in which the wound is found [83, 84].

Investigations on DFU wounds are limited by appearance to obtain tissue biopsies. The wounds secrete liquid, which can be obtained in a non-invasive way for the patient, solving the problem a little for future investigations. The use of wound secretion is supported by previous investigations, where a high bacterial count has been demonstrated, and this of course resulting in poor wound healing [85]. High concentrations of MMP-9 have been demonstrated, giving a prediction that would lead to poor healing in DFU. Although the mechanism that generates the increase of MMP-9 is not yet known, it is associated with the inflammatory syndrome, since MMP-9 is being synthesized by neutrophils and macrophages [86]. It has been found in previous studies that the high bacterial count in the wound despite the absence of infection is indicative of poor wound healing [85]. Generating the hypothesis about a high bacterial count and high concentrations of MMP is also related to poor healing. It has also been demonstrated a statistically significant relationship between the MMP-1/TIMP-1 and the favorable healing [87]. MMP-1 is the main responsible for healing collagenase-related due to the benefit it brings to complete the proliferative phase; this has shown that degradation of collagen I is required for keratinocyte migration, which involves re-epidermization [24, 88]. Other studies of MMP have studied the role of MMP-2; however, it is not yet clear, due to variations in expression or concentration levels. This proposes the role of MMP-2 at least in chronic wounds, because MMP-2 is known to be synthesized by fibroblasts that are secreted in the proliferative phase where inflammation predominates [89, 90].

2.8. MMPs and topical and biologic therapies for DFU

It is reported that the dynamic changes on the content and activity of MMP-2 and/or TIMP-2, are secreted by fibroblasts majorly, play much essential parts in the normal healings, especially during the midterm and later phases, including accelerating revascularization, granulation tissues regeneration as well as the connective tissues reformation and safeguarding the normal dermis to some extent [91]. Owning to the decreased content and/or activity of growth factors and the disturbed balance of MMPs/TIMPs system, which results in excessive solvent activity and then reduced content or damaged structure of the growth factors and ECMs, the diabetic cutaneous ulcers are always poorly healed. MMP-2 is found to be excessively generated while TIMP-2 is deficiently secreted in diabetic chronic wounds, and the pathologic imbalance may bring about retarded progress of tissue regeneration and revascularization [86]. The efficacy of autologous platelet-rich gel (APG) on refractory wounds in the healing mechanism is recognized [92, 93] including upregulating the content of many growth factors and releasing antibacterial peptides [94]. Furthermore, in some basic researches, TGF-β1 has been reported to inhibit the generation of MMP-2 by depressing its genetic transcription and enhance that of TIMP-2 meanwhile [5]. In preliminary clinical studies, the local concentration of TGF-β1 increases after APG treatment [95]. This has been proven and reported, where APG treatment may suppress the expression of MMP-2 and promote that of TIMP-2 in the diabetic chronic refractory cutaneous wounds and furthermore decrease the ratio of the MMP-2/TIMP-2, and TGF-β1 may be related to these effects [96].

The photobiomodulation (PBM) is a noninvasive form of light therapy for wound healing, whereby several biological, chemical and cellular processes are stimulated to speed up healing; investigations carried out demonstrated PBM to enhance wound healing [97]. The biostimulatory effect of PBM in the near infrared (NIR) range modulates wound healing events in various cells. This generates an increased collagen activity twofold, increased MMP-2 activity, upregulated MMP-1 and TIMP-2 expression and down regulated MMP-2 and IL-1β [98]. These findings are of therapeutic importance in situations with depleted smooth cells, weakened ECM and increased pro-inflammatory markers as major pathological components. The PBM is able to alter the expression of MMPs in diabetic wounds and enhance collagen production; however, experiments done on human skin demonstrated variations in gene expression in the fibroblasts [99]. Yadav et al. (2014) found that PBM altered 49 genes involved in the ECM in vitro, with genes in a diabetic wounded cell model mostly downregulated, among which were MMP-1, MMP-2, MMP-8, MMP-12, MMP-14 and MMP-16 [75]. PBM is known for its stimulatory effects and promotes MMP activity and gene expression; hence maintaining a dynamic balance between the proteolytic activity and degradation could be a target for therapeutic advancement [99]. However, its effect on various matrix proteins still needs to be further understood.

3. Conclusions

In the course of the regeneration of a lesion, degradation in the formation of blood vessels is necessary, also so that there is adequate cell migration and a proteolysis of the ECM to obtain a remodeling of granulation tissue. Consequently, the degradation is under a precise and strict control, where the loss of homeostasis between ECM deposition and proteolysis results in a significant failure in wound healing, as occurs in DFUs. MMPs play a significant role in tissue remodeling; their role in normal and abnormal wound healing is not well characterized. The MMPs are known for degradation of the ECM and have been shown to be upregulated in most pathologies; in the case of DFUs, they have been recognized as predicting and its expression may show alterations in the tissues, serum, plasma or fluid of wounds identify the mechanisms involved in wound healing and thereby to intervene proactively to prevent the normal wound from becoming chronic and later in diabetic ulcer or amputation and if this progress may lead to death.

Acknowledgements

This work was funded in part by CONACyT: INFR-2014-01-225520, INFR-2015-01-254106, PDCPN-2015-01-63, SEP-CONACYT-CB-2015-258316 and SS/IMSS/ISSSTE-CONACYT-2016-01-273144. The first author wants to thank the CONACyT doctorate scholarship, with scholarship holder number 695781.

Author details

Claudia Castruita-De la Rosa[1,2], Idalia Garza-Veloz[1,2*], Edith Cardenas-Vargas[1,3], Rodrigo Castañeda-Miranda[2], Luis O. Solis-Sanchez[2], Jose M. Ortiz-Rodriguez[2], Hector R. Vega-Carrillo[2], Maria R. Martinez-Blanco[2], Virginia Flores-Morales[4], Gloria P. Hernandez-Delgadillo[5], Jose I. Badillo-Almaráz[1] and Margarita L. Martinez-Fierro[1,2*]

*Address all correspondence to: margaritamf@uaz.edu.mx and idaliagv@uaz.edu.mx

1 Molecular Medicine Laboratory, Unidad Académica de Medicina Humana y Ciencias de la Salud, Universidad Autónoma de Zacatecas, Zacatecas, México

2 Centro de Innovación Tecnológica e Industrial, Unidad Académica de Ingeniería Eléctrica, Universidad Autónoma de Zacatecas, Zacatecas, México

3 Hospital General Zacatecas "Luz González Cosío", Servicios de Salud de Zacatecas, Zacatecas, México

4 Laboratorio de Síntesis Asimétrica y Bioenergética (LSAyB), Universidad Autónoma de Zacatecas, Zacatecas, México

5 Laboratorio de Investigación en Farmacología, Universidad Autónoma de Zacatecas, Zacatecas, México

References

[1] Association AD. Diagnosis and classification of diabetes. In: Diabetes Care. Vol. 33. American Diabetes Association; 2010. pp. 562-569

http://dx.doi.org/10.5772/intechopen.71725

[2] Moffarah AS, Al Mohajer M, Hurwitz BL, Armstrong DG. Skin and soft tissue infections. Microbiology Spectrum. 2016;**4**(4):1-16

[3] Diabetes FId. Atlas de la Diabetes de la FID. 7th ed. International Diabetes Federation; 2015

[4] Chadwick P, Edmonds M, McCardle J, Armstrong D. International Best Practice Guidelines: Wound Management in Diabetic Foot Ulcers. Wounds International; 2013. pp. 1-27

[5] Armstrong DG, Jude EB. The role of matrix metalloproteinases in wound healing. Journal of the American Podiatric Medical Association. 2002;**92**(1):12-18

[6] Patterson BC, Sang QA. Angiostatin-converting enzyme activities of human matrilysin (MMP-7) and gelatinase B/type IV collagenase (MMP-9). The Journal of Biological Chemistry. 1997;**272**(46):28823-28825

[7] Rohani MG, Parks WC. Matrix remodeling by MMPs during wound repair. Matrix Biology: Journal of the International Society for Matrix Biology. 2015;**44-46**:113-121

[8] Khokha R, Murthy A, Weiss A. Metalloproteinases and their natural inhibitors in inflammation and immunity. Nature Reviews Immunology. 2013;**13**(9):649-665

[9] Overall CM, Lopez-Otin C. Strategies for MMP inhibition in cancer: Innovations for the post-trial era. Nature Reviews Cancer. 2002;**2**(9):657-672

[10] Egeblad M, Werb Z. New functions for the matrix metalloproteinases in cancer progression. Nature Reviews Cancer. 2002;**2**(3):161-174

[11] Sternlicht MD, Werb Z. How matrix metalloproteinases regulate cell behavior. Annual Review of Cell and Developmental Biology. 2001;**17**:463-516

[12] Murphy G. Tissue inhibitors of metalloproteinases. Genome Biology. 2011;**12**(11):233

[13] Hernandez-Barrantes S, Toth M, Bernardo MM, Yurkova M, Gervasi DC, Raz Y, Sang QA, Fridman R. Binding of active (57 kDa) membrane type 1-matrix metalloproteinase (MT1-MMP) to tissue inhibitor of metalloproteinase (TIMP)-2 regulates MT1-MMP processing and pro-MMP-2 activation. The Journal of Biological Chemistry. 2000;**275**(16): 12080-12089

[14] Brew K, Nagase H. The tissue inhibitors of metalloproteinases (TIMPs): An ancient family with structural and functional diversity. Biochimica et Biophysica Acta. 2010; **1803**(1):55-71

[15] Rivera S, Khrestchatisky M, Kaczmarek L, Rosenberg GA, Jaworski DM. Metzincin proteases and their inhibitors: Foes or friends in nervous system physiology? The Journal of neuroscience: The official journal of the Society for Neuroscience. 2010;**30**(46): 15337-15357

[16] Nagase H, Visse R, Murphy G. Structure and function of matrix metalloproteinases and TIMPs. Cardiovascular Research. 2006;**69**(3):562-573

[17] Lemaitre V, D'Armiento J. Matrix metalloproteinases in development and disease. Birth Defects Research Part C, Embryo Today: Reviews. 2006;**78**(1):1-10

[18] Park JH, Jeong YJ, Park KK, Cho HJ, Chung IK, Min KS, Kim M, Lee KG, Yeo JH, Chang YC. Melittin suppresses PMA-induced tumor cell invasion by inhibiting NF-kappaB and AP-1-dependent MMP-9 expression. Molecules and Cells. 2010;**29**(2):209-215

[19] Westermarck J, Kahari VM. Regulation of matrix metalloproteinase expression in tumor invasion. FASEB Journal: Official Publication of the Federation of American Societies for Experimental Biology. 1999;**13**(8):781-792

[20] Lu J, Guo JH, XL T, Zhang C, Zhao M, Zhang QW, Gao FH. Tiron inhibits UVB-induced AP-1 binding sites transcriptional activation on MMP-1 and MMP-3 promoters by MAPK signaling pathway in human dermal fibroblasts. PLoS One. 2016;**11**(8):e0159998

[21] Lohi J, Lehti K, Valtanen H, Parks WC, Keski-Oja J. Structural analysis and promoter characterization of the human membrane-type matrix metalloproteinase-1 (MT1-MMP) gene. Gene. 2000;**242**(1-2):75-86

[22] Visse R, Nagase H. Matrix metalloproteinases and tissue inhibitors of metalloproteinases: Structure, function, and biochemistry. Circulation Research. 2003;**92**(8):827-839

[23] Lijnen HR. Plasmin and matrix metalloproteinases in vascular remodeling. Thrombosis and Haemostasis. 2001;**86**(1):324-333

[24] Pilcher BK, Dumin JA, Sudbeck BD, Krane SM, Welgus HG, Parks WC. The activity of collagenase-1 is required for keratinocyte migration on a type I collagen matrix. The Journal of Cell Biology. 1997;**137**(6):1445-1457

[25] Chang M. Restructuring of the extracellular matrix in diabetic wounds and healing: A perspective. Pharmacological Research. 2016;**107**:243-248

[26] Ravanti L, Kahari VM. Matrix metalloproteinases in wound repair (review). International Journal of Molecular Medicine. 2000;**6**(4):391-407

[27] Robson MC, Steed DL, Franz MG. Wound healing: Biologic features and approaches to maximize healing trajectories. Current Problems in Surgery. 2001;**38**(2):72-140

[28] Heng MC. Wound healing in adult skin: Aiming for perfect regeneration. International Journal of Dermatology. 2011;**50**(9):1058-1066

[29] Woo YC, Park SS, Subieta AR, Brennan TJ. Changes in tissue pH and temperature after incision indicate acidosis may contribute to postoperative pain. Anesthesiology. 2004; **101**(2):468-475

[30] Werner S, Grose R. Regulation of wound healing by growth factors and cytokines. Physiological Reviews. 2003;**83**(3):835-870

[31] Heldin CH, Westermark B. Mechanism of action and in vivo role of platelet-derived growth factor. Physiological Reviews. 1999;**79**(4):1283-1316

[32] Momota Y, Suzuki N, Kasuya Y, Kobayashi T, Mizoguchi M, Yokoyama F, Nomizu M, Shinkai H, Iwasaki T, Utani A. Laminin alpha3 LG4 module induces keratinocyte migration:

Involvement of matrix metalloproteinase-9. Journal of Receptor and Signal Transduction Research. 2005;**25**(1):1-17

[33] Giannelli G, Falk-Marzillier J, Schiraldi O, Stetler-Stevenson WG, Quaranta V. Induction of cell migration by matrix metalloprotease-2 cleavage of laminin-5. Science. 1997;**277**(5323): 225-228

[34] Koshikawa N, Giannelli G, Cirulli V, Miyazaki K, Quaranta V. Role of cell surface metalloprotease MT1-MMP in epithelial cell migration over laminin-5. The Journal of Cell Biology. 2000;**148**(3):615-624

[35] Makela M, Larjava H, Pirila E, Maisi P, Salo T, Sorsa T, Uitto VJ. Matrix metalloproteinase 2 (gelatinase A) is related to migration of keratinocytes. Experimental Cell Research. 1999;**251**(1):67-78

[36] McCawley LJ, O'Brien P, Hudson LG. Epidermal growth factor (EGF)- and scatter factor/hepatocyte growth factor (SF/HGF)-mediated keratinocyte migration is coincident with induction of matrix metalloproteinase (MMP)-9. Journal of Cellular Physiology. 1998;**176**(2):255-265

[37] Branco da Cunha C, Klumpers DD, Li WA, Koshy ST, Weaver JC, Chaudhuri O, Granja PL, Mooney DJ. Influence of the stiffness of three-dimensional alginate/collagen-I interpenetrating networks on fibroblast biology. Biomaterials. 2014;**35**(32):8927-8936

[38] Jacinto A, Martinez-Arias A, Martin P. Mechanisms of epithelial fusion and repair. Nature Cell Biology. 2001;**3**(5):E117-E123

[39] Hinz B. Formation and function of the myofibroblast during tissue repair. The Journal of Investigative Dermatology. 2007;**127**(3):526-537

[40] Wysocki AB, Staiano-Coico L, Grinnell F. Wound fluid from chronic leg ulcers contains elevated levels of metalloproteinases MMP-2 and MMP-9. The Journal of Investigative Dermatology. 1993;**101**(1):64-68

[41] Takeo M, Lee W, Ito M. Wound healing and skin regeneration. Cold Spring Harbor Perspectives in Medicine. 2015;**5**(1):a023267

[42] Rosinczuk J, Taradaj J, Dymarek R, Sopel M. Mechanoregulation of wound healing and skin homeostasis. BioMed Research International. 2016;**2016**:3943481

[43] Saarialho-Kere UK. Patterns of matrix metalloproteinase and TIMP expression in chronic ulcers. Archives of Dermatological Research. 1998;**290**(Suppl):S47-S54

[44] Arpino V, Brock M, Gill SE. The role of TIMPs in regulation of extracellular matrix proteolysis. Matrix Biology: Journal of the International Society for Matrix Biology. 2015; **44-46**:247-254

[45] Sadowski T, Dietrich S, Muller M, Havlickova B, Schunck M, Proksch E, Muller MS, Sedlacek R. Matrix metalloproteinase-19 expression in normal and diseased skin: Dysregulation by epidermal proliferation. The Journal of Investigative Dermatology. 2003;**121**(5):989-996

[46] Inoue M, Kratz G, Haegerstrand A, Stahle-Backdahl M. Collagenase expression is rapidly induced in wound-edge keratinocytes after acute injury in human skin, persists during healing, and stops at re-epithelialization. The Journal of Investigative Dermatology. 1995;**104**(4):479-483

[47] Sudbeck BD, Pilcher BK, Welgus HG, Parks WC. Induction and repression of collagenase-1 by keratinocytes is controlled by distinct components of different extracellular matrix compartments. The Journal of Biological Chemistry. 1997;**272**(35):22103-22110

[48] Di Colandrea T, Wang L, Wille J, D'Armiento J, Chada KK. Epidermal expression of collagenase delays wound-healing in transgenic mice. The Journal of Investigative Dermatology. 1998;**111**(6):1029-1033

[49] Ravanti L, Toriseva M, Penttinen R, Crombleholme T, Foschi M, Han J, Kahari VM. Expression of human collagenase-3 (MMP-13) by fetal skin fibroblasts is induced by transforming growth factor beta via p38 mitogen-activated protein kinase. FASEB Journal: Official Publication of the Federation of American Societies for Experimental Biology. 2001;**15**(6):1098-1100

[50] Toriseva MJ, Ala-aho R, Karvinen J, Baker AH, Marjomaki VS, Heino J, Kahari VM. Collagenase-3 (MMP-13) enhances remodeling of three-dimensional collagen and promotes survival of human skin fibroblasts. The Journal of Investigative Dermatology. 2007;**127**(1):49-59

[51] Nissinen L, Kahari VM. Matrix metalloproteinases in inflammation. Biochimica et Biophysica Acta. 2014;**1840**(8):2571-2580

[52] Holmbeck K, Bianco P, Caterina J, Yamada S, Kromer M, Kuznetsov SA, Mankani M, Robey PG, Poole AR, Pidoux I, et al. MT1-MMP-deficient mice develop dwarfism, osteopenia, arthritis, and connective tissue disease due to inadequate collagen turnover. Cell. 1999;**99**(1):81-92

[53] Rechardt O, Elomaa O, Vaalamo M, Paakkonen K, Jahkola T, Hook-Nikanne J, Hembry RM, Hakkinen L, Kere J, Saarialho-Kere U. Stromelysin-2 is upregulated during normal wound repair and is induced by cytokines. The Journal of Investigative Dermatology. 2000;**115**(5):778-787

[54] Chen W, Fu X, Ge S, Sun T, Sheng Z. Differential expression of matrix metalloproteinases and tissue-derived inhibitors of metalloproteinase in fetal and adult skins. The International Journal of Biochemistry & Cell Biology. 2007;**39**(5):997-1005

[55] Mirastschijski U, Impola U, Jahkola T, Karlsmark T, AG MS, Saarialho-Kere U. Ectopic localization of matrix metalloproteinase-9 in chronic cutaneous wounds. Human Pathology. 2002;**33**(3):355-364

[56] Mohan R, Chintala SK, Jung JC, Villar WV, McCabe F, Russo LA, Lee Y, McCarthy BE, Wollenberg KR, Jester JV, et al. Matrix metalloproteinase gelatinase B (MMP-9) coordinates and effects epithelial regeneration. The Journal of Biological Chemistry. 2002; **277**(3):2065-2072

[57] Bergers G, Brekken R, McMahon G, TH V, Itoh T, Tamaki K, Tanzawa K, Thorpe P, Itohara S, Werb Z, et al. Matrix metalloproteinase-9 triggers the angiogenic switch during carcinogenesis. Nature Cell Biology. 2000;**2**(10):737-744

[58] Chun TH, Sabeh F, Ota I, Murphy H, McDonagh KT, Holmbeck K, Birkedal-Hansen H, Allen ED, Weiss SJ. MT1-MMP-dependent neovessel formation within the confines of the three-dimensional extracellular matrix. The Journal of Cell Biology. 2004;**167**(4):757-767

[59] Impola U, Toriseva M, Suomela S, Jeskanen L, Hieta N, Jahkola T, Grenman R, Kahari VM, Saarialho-Kere U. Matrix metalloproteinase-19 is expressed by proliferating epithelium but disappears with neoplastic dedifferentiation. International Journal of Cancer. 2003;**103**(6):709-716

[60] Lazaro JL, Izzo V, Meaume S, Davies AH, Lobmann R, Uccioli L. Elevated levels of matrix metalloproteinases and chronic wound healing: An updated review of clinical evidence. Journal of Wound Care. 2016;**25**(5):277-287

[61] Nwomeh BC, Liang HX, Cohen IK, Yager DR. MMP-8 is the predominant collagenase in healing wounds and nonhealing ulcers. The Journal of Surgical Research. 1999; **81**(2):189-195

[62] Rayment EA, Upton Z, Shooter GK. Increased matrix metalloproteinase-9 (MMP-9) activity observed in chronic wound fluid is related to the clinical severity of the ulcer. The British Journal of Dermatology. 2008;**158**(5):951-961

[63] Lobmann R, Ambrosch A, Schultz G, Waldmann K, Schiweck S, Lehnert H. Expression of matrix-metalloproteinases and their inhibitors in the wounds of diabetic and non-diabetic patients. Diabetologia. 2002;**45**(7):1011-1016

[64] Krisp C, Jacobsen F, McKay MJ, Molloy MP, Steinstraesser L, Wolters DA. Proteome analysis reveals antiangiogenic environments in chronic wounds of diabetes mellitus type 2 patients. Proteomics. 2013;**13**(17):2670-2681

[65] Barone EJ, Yager DR, Pozez AL, Olutoye OO, Crossland MC, Diegelmann RF, Cohen IK. Interleukin-1alpha and collagenase activity are elevated in chronic wounds. Plastic and Reconstructive Surgery. 1998;**102**(4):1023-1027 discussion 1028-1029

[66] de Oliveira RR, Lemos A, de Castro Silveira PV, da Silva RJ, de Moraes SR. Alterations of tendons in patients with diabetes mellitus: A systematic review. Diabetic Medicine: A Journal of the British Diabetic Association. 2011;**28**(8):886-895

[67] Izzo V, Meloni M, Vainieri E, Giurato L, Ruotolo V, Uccioli L. High matrix metalloproteinase levels are associated with dermal graft failure in diabetic foot ulcers. The International Journal of Lower Extremity Wounds. 2014;**13**(3):191-196

[68] Kadoglou NP, Daskalopoulou SS, Perrea D, Liapis CD. Matrix metalloproteinases and diabetic vascular complications. Angiology. 2005;**56**(2):173-189

[69] Ban CR, Twigg SM. Fibrosis in diabetes complications: Pathogenic mechanisms and circulating and urinary markers. Vascular Health and Risk Management. 2008;**4**(3):575-596

[70] Mendias CL, Gumucio JP, Davis ME, Bromley CW, Davis CS, Brooks SV. Transforming growth factor-beta induces skeletal muscle atrophy and fibrosis through the induction of atrogin-1 and scleraxis. Muscle & Nerve. 2012;**45**(1):55-59

[71] Dinh T, Tecilazich F, Kafanas A, Doupis J, Gnardellis C, Leal E, Tellechea A, Pradhan L, Lyons TE, Giurini JM, et al. Mechanisms involved in the development and healing of diabetic foot ulceration. Diabetes. 2012;**61**(11):2937-2947

[72] Martins VL, Caley M, O'Toole EA. Matrix metalloproteinases and epidermal wound repair. Cell and Tissue Research. 2013;**351**(2):255-268

[73] Chung AW, Hsiang YN, Matzke LA, McManus BM, van Breemen C, Okon EB. Reduced expression of vascular endothelial growth factor paralleled with the increased angiostatin expression resulting from the upregulated activities of matrix metalloproteinase-2 and -9 in human type 2 diabetic arterial vasculature. Circulation Research. 2006;**99**(2): 140-148

[74] Death AK, Fisher EJ, McGrath KC, Yue DK. High glucose alters matrix metalloproteinase expression in two key vascular cells: Potential impact on atherosclerosis in diabetes. Atherosclerosis. 2003;**168**(2):263-269

[75] Yadav SS, Singh MK, Dwivedi P, Mandal RK, Usman K, Khattri S, Pant KK. Significance of impaired serum gelatinases activities in metabolic syndrome. Toxicology International. 2014;**21**(1):107-111

[76] Li Z, Guo S, Yao F, Zhang Y, Li T. Increased ratio of serum matrix metalloproteinase-9 against TIMP-1 predicts poor wound healing in diabetic foot ulcers. Journal of Diabetes and its Complications. 2013;**27**(4):380-382

[77] Menghini R, Uccioli L, Vainieri E, Pecchioli C, Casagrande V, Stoehr R, Cardellini M, Porzio O, Rizza S, Federici M. Expression of tissue inhibitor of metalloprotease 3 is reduced in ischemic but not neuropathic ulcers from patients with type 2 diabetes mellitus. Acta Diabetologica. 2013;**50**(6):907-910

[78] Lopez-Lopez N, Gonzalez-Curiel I, Trevino-Santa Cruz MB, Rivas-Santiago B, Trujillo-Paez V, Enciso-Moreno JA, Serrano CJ. Expression and vitamin D-mediated regulation of matrix metalloproteinases (MMPs) and tissue inhibitors of metalloproteinases (TIMPs) in healthy skin and in diabetic foot ulcers. Archives of Dermatological Research. 2014;**306**(9):809-821

[79] Serra R, Buffone G, Falcone D, Molinari V, Scaramuzzino M, Gallelli L, de Franciscis S. Chronic venous leg ulcers are associated with high levels of metalloproteinases-9 and neutrophil gelatinase-associated lipocalin. Wound Repair and Regeneration: Official Publication of the Wound Healing Society [and] The European Tissue Repair Society. 2013;**21**(3):395-401

[80] Amato B, Coretti G, Compagna R, Amato M, Buffone G, Gigliotti D, Grande R, Serra R, de Franciscis S. Role of matrix metalloproteinases in non-healing venous ulcers. International Wound Journal. 2015;**12**(6):641-645

[81] Burrow JW, Koch JA, Chuang HH, Zhong W, Dean DD, Sylvia VL. Nitric oxide donors selectively reduce the expression of matrix metalloproteinases-8 and -9 by human diabetic skin fibroblasts. The Journal of Surgical Research. 2007;**140**(1):90-98

[82] Uccioli L, Izzo V, Meloni M, Vainieri E, Ruotolo V, Giurato L. Non-healing foot ulcers in diabetic patients: General and local interfering conditions and management options with advanced wound dressings. Journal of Wound Care. 2015;**24**(4 Suppl):35-42

[83] Madlener M, Parks WC, Werner S. Matrix metalloproteinases (MMPs) and their physiological inhibitors (TIMPs) are differentially expressed during excisional skin wound repair. Experimental Cell Research. 1998;**242**(1):201-210

[84] Lobmann R, Zemlin C, Motzkau M, Reschke K, Lehnert H. Expression of matrix metalloproteinases and growth factors in diabetic foot wounds treated with a protease absorbent dressing. Journal of Diabetes and its Complications. 2006;**20**(5):329-335

[85] Xu L, McLennan SV, Lo L, Natfaji A, Bolton T, Liu Y, Twigg SM, Yue DK. Bacterial load predicts healing rate in neuropathic diabetic foot ulcers. Diabetes Care. 2007;**30**(2):378-380

[86] Falanga V. Wound healing and its impairment in the diabetic foot. Lancet. 2005; **366**(9498):1736-1743

[87] Muller M, Trocme C, Lardy B, Morel F, Halimi S, Benhamou PY. Matrix metalloproteinases and diabetic foot ulcers: The ratio of MMP-1 to TIMP-1 is a predictor of wound healing. Diabetic Medicine: A Journal of the British Diabetic Association. 2008;**25**(4):419-426

[88] Stamenkovic I. Extracellular matrix remodelling: The role of matrix metalloproteinases. The Journal of Pathology. 2003;**200**(4):448-464

[89] Yager DR, Zhang LY, Liang HX, Diegelmann RF, Cohen IK. Wound fluids from human pressure ulcers contain elevated matrix metalloproteinase levels and activity compared to surgical wound fluids. The Journal of Investigative Dermatology. 1996;**107**(5):743-748

[90] Vaalamo M, Mattila L, Johansson N, Kariniemi AL, Karjalainen-Lindsberg ML, Kahari VM, Saarialho-Kere U. Distinct populations of stromal cells express collagenase-3 (MMP-13) and collagenase-1 (MMP-1) in chronic ulcers but not in normally healing wounds. The Journal of Investigative Dermatology. 1997;**109**(1):96-101

[91] Soo C, Shaw WW, Zhang X, Longaker MT, Howard EW, Ting K. Differential expression of matrix metalloproteinases and their tissue-derived inhibitors in cutaneous wound repair. Plastic and Reconstructive Surgery. 2000;**105**(2):638-647

[92] Yuan NB, Wang C, Wang Y, Yu TT, Shu SQ, Liu M, Ran XW. The preliminary application of autologous platelet-rich gel used to treat refractory diabetic dermal ulcer. Sichuan da xue xue bao Yi xue ban = Journal of Sichuan University Medical Science Edition. 2007;**38**(5):900-903

[93] Driver VR, Hanft J, Fylling CP, Beriou JM. A prospective, randomized, controlled trial of autologous platelet-rich plasma gel for the treatment of diabetic foot ulcers. Ostomy/ Wound Management. 2006;**52**(6):68-70, 72, 74 passim

[94] Chen L, Wang C, Liu H, Liu G, Ran X. Antibacterial effect of autologous platelet-rich gel derived from subjects with diabetic dermal ulcers in vitro. Journal of Diabetes Research. 2013;**2013**:269527

[95] Jude EB, Blakytny R, Bulmer J, Boulton AJ, Ferguson MW. Transforming growth factor-beta 1, 2, 3 and receptor type I and II in diabetic foot ulcers. Diabetic Medicine: A Journal of the British Diabetic Association. 2002;**19**(6):440-447

[96] Li L, Chen D, Wang C, Liu G, Ran X. The effect of autologous platelet-rich gel on the dynamic changes of the matrix metalloproteinase-2 and tissue inhibitor of metalloproteinase-2 expression in the diabetic chronic refractory cutaneous ulcers. Journal of Diabetes Research. 2015;**2015**:954701

[97] Primo FL, de Paula LB, de Siqueira-Moura MP, Tedesco AC. Photobiostimulation on wound healing treatment by ClAlPc-nanoemulsion from a multiple-wavelength portable light source on a 3D-human stem cell dermal equivalent. Current Medicinal Chemistry. 2012;**19**(30):5157-5163

[98] Gavish L, Perez L, Gertz SD. Low-level laser irradiation modulates matrix metalloproteinase activity and gene expression in porcine aortic smooth muscle cells. Lasers in Surgery and Medicine. 2006;**38**(8):779-786

[99] Ayuk SM, Houreld NN, Abrahamse H. Laser irradiation alters the expression profile of genes involved in the extracellular matrix in vitro. International Journal of Photoenergy. 2014;**17**:1-17